The Gout Diet Cookbook

Low-Purine Diet Next Level and Tasty Recipes and a Guide to Natural Foods with

Anti-Inflammatory Properties

Harlan Josh Walsh

Table of Contents

CHAPTER 7:

CHAPTER 8:

CHAPTER 12:

CHAPTER 13:

CHAPTER 14:

INTRODUCTION

I have been on a purine-restricted diet for fourteen years. I have consistently sought out any research on gout, trying to apply it to my personal experience. I believe I have finally found an effective diet that helps me, and I am eager to share my experience with you.

Understanding and following the diet is essential for those with hyperuricemia and gout. A low-purine diet is a necessity for those with elevated uric acid levels, which can lead to gout and kidney stones. The author's desire for a healthier and more energetic life is at the heart of the pages of *The Gout Diet Cookbook*.

I believe that everyone who is facing the problem of gout will find in my book tips and inspiration on how to organize their diet for the greater benefit of their body. Now, let's embark on our culinary journey!

Chapter 1:

The Role of Purines in the Body and Their Impact

Purines are natural substances in the body's cells and virtually all foods. They are metabolized into uric acid, an antioxidant that helps prevent damage caused by active oxygen species.

A continuous supply of uric acid is vital for protecting human blood vessels.

Frequent and high intake of purine-rich foods can increase serum uric acid levels, which can lead to gout and also potentially increase the risk of cardiovascular disease.

There is a recommended daily intake of dietary purines to prevent gout and hyperuricemia. It is less than 400 mg. Purine-rich foods include animal meats and organ meats, fish meats, other seafood, and yeast.

Four purine bases exist (adenine, guanine, hypoxanthine, and xanthine). Adenine and guanine are mainly found in cereals, beans, soybean products, seaweeds, dairy products, mushrooms, and vegetables.

Most animal meats and processed meat items, except giblets, contain a high ratio of hypoxanthine. Fresh fish meat also contains a high ratio of hypoxanthine. Many mollusks contain adenine and guanine.

For gout and hyperuricemia patients, the total purine intake and the specific types of purines consumed, especially hypoxanthine, are important considerations.

Hypoxanthine has a more substantial effect than other purines. Therefore, foods that contain a large amount of total purines and a high ratio of hypoxanthine are considered the most significant dietary risk factors for developing gout and should be consumed in moderation. Acute purine intake also increases the risk of recurrent gout attacks by almost fivefold.

Chapter 2:
How I Came to My Current Diet

Fourteen years ago, I started a diet that restricts consumption to no more than 100 grams of meat or seafood twice a week. It also eliminates foods very high in oxalates and acidic substances.

However, two years ago, due to deteriorating health, I decided to try a vegan diet. Initially, it was challenging to give up animal-derived products. It took not just a month but nearly three for my habits to change completely. After this time, the desire to frequently consume meat, fish, eggs, and animal fats has disappeared.

Listening to my body, I realized I was on the right path. I lost weight and felt better. I didn't count calories. I've learned and will stick with eating plenty of seeds and handful of nuts. Unfortunately, I cannot eat as many legumes as needed.

I had to make changes to my diet after ten months on a vegan diet.

I've come to the conclusion that it's best for me to consume:

- ✓ Meat twice a month, no more than 50–100 g
- ✓ Fish three times a month, no more than 50–100 g
- ✓ Other seafood once a month, no more than 50 g
- ✓ Meat or seafood no more than once every five days
- ✓ I still exclude foods with very high oxalate content and acidic foods.
- ✓ A little cheese or plain yogurt every day

- ✓ Eggs should only be used in baked goods (in moderation)
- ✓ I use only vegetable oils, primarily olive oil
- ✓ I buy a variety of vegetable oils. I take a teaspoon of oil in the morning to improve my health.
- ✓ I've also limited my salt and sugar intake. I try to consume no more than a teaspoon of salt daily and seven teaspoons of sugar.

Sucrose, or "table sugar," is 50% fructose and 50% glucose. I don't add sugar to my drinks, only to my baked goods, which are my stress reliever. I am gradually reducing the amount of sugar in it. I already use no more than half a cup of sugar in the baking recipes in this book.

With this diet, I can afford higher-quality meat, wild fish, seafood, cheese, and extra virgin olive oil. I don't count calories. I call it the "low-purine diet: the next level."

I have read that animal proteins, unlike plant proteins, can lead to increased acidity in the body. They encourage it to leach calcium from the bones, which can lead to fractures and increased calcium levels in the urine. Additionally, animal proteins can contribute to the formation of kidney stones.

I'm glad I consume a modest amount of animal proteins and fats. I've long eliminated acidic foods from my diet, including vinegar and products very high in oxalic acid (for the prevention of kidney stones). Salts from oxalic acid are called oxalates.

I enjoy chia seeds, flax seeds, sesame paste, tofu, chickpeas, amaranth, and quinoa. One hundred grams of unhulled sesame seeds contain 989 mg (99%RDA) of calcium. Hopefully, I'll get used to this product.

One hundred grams of chia seeds contain calcium 631 mg (63%RDA). Chia seeds soaked in water help my stomach.
I soak all legumes (chickpeas overnight) and beans for 24 hours. I change the water twice for chickpeas and three or four times for beans. This treatment helps to reduce phytic acid (it interferes with mineral absorption). I use canned legumes if I don't have time, but I always rinse them.

I sometimes buy iron, vitamin B12, D3, Omega-3. To reduce purines in foods, I boil them and don't use broth as it has a lot of purines. After boiling or pouring boiling water over soy meat, I thoroughly squeeze it to reduce the purine content. I eat this product no more than once a week.

I cook more than needed and freeze the leftovers. It's not every day I have time to cook, and there is more variety on the table.

I follow the doctor's recommendations and take my medications when needed.

My method of fighting the disease is constant daily prevention.

Chapter 3:
Review of Foods that Help Maintain the Diet

Two key factors need to be considered. The first is the total amount of purines in the food, and the second is which types of purine bases it contains. Consuming foods that contain more than 200 mg per 3.53 ounces or 100 g of purines, especially those with high levels of hypoxanthine, is considered a high risk for hyperuricemia. This group includes animal meats, fish, and some shrimp.

The specified amount of purines is 3.53 ounces or 100 grams.

Most grains, legumes, and soy products contain less than 50 mg of purines. Dried soybeans contain more purines than other beans, at 172.5 mg, while raw green soybeans contain much less at 47.9 mg. All soy products, including tofu and soy milk, contain less than 50 mg of purines.

Although wakame has 262 mg and nori has 591.7 mg of purines, they are dried and very lightweight, and only a small amount is used in cooking. Parsley contains 288.9 mg of total purines. Like seaweed, parsley is used in small quantities (no more than 2 grams) in cooking or as a garnish.

Dried shiitake mushrooms contain 379.5 mg of purines—much more than fresh ones, which have 20.8 mg.

Young spinach leaves contain 172 mg of purines—much more than mature spinach leaves, which have 51.5 mg. Broccoli sprouts contain 129.6 mg of purines—much more than regular broccoli, which has 70 mg.

Meat That Contains Fewer Purines than Other Parts

In 3.53 ounces or 100 grams:

Beef

- ✓ Beef brisket (hypoxanthine 49 mg), total purine content
- ✓ 79 mg.
- ✓ Beef ribloin (hypoxanthine 39.5 mg), total purine content 74 mg.
- ✓ Beef tenderloin (hypoxanthine 64 mg), total purine content 98.4 mg.
- ✓ Shoulder sirloin (hypoxanthine 55.8 mg), total purine content 90 mg.

Chicken

- ✓ Chicken buttocks (hypoxanthine 23.2 mg), total purine content 68.8 mg.
- ✓ Chicken leg (hypoxanthine 76.2 mg), total purine content 122.9 mg.

Pork

- ✓ Pork neck (hypoxanthine 43.6 mg), total purine content 70.5 mg.
- ✓ Pork ribs (hypoxanthine 51.7 mg), total purine content
- ✓ 75.8 mg.
- ✓ Pork shoulder (hypoxanthine 53.1 mg), total purine content 81.4 mg.
- ✓ Pork sirloin (hypoxanthine 61.2 mg), total purine content 90.9 mg.

Lamb

- ✓ Lamb (hypoxanthine 87.5 mg), total purine content
- ✓ 127.5 mg.

Turkey

- ✓ Turkey (hypoxanthine 41.2 mg), total purine content 79 mg.
- ✓ Turkey skin contains 150 mg.

Meat That Contains More Purines

Chicken

- ✓ Chicken breast (hypoxanthine 98.4 mg), total purine content 141.2 mg.
- ✓ Chicken white meat (hypoxanthine 110.2 mg), total purine content 153.9 mg.
- ✓ Chicken wing (hypoxanthine 92.5 mg), total purine content 137.5 mg.

Fish

- ✓ Salmon (hypoxanthine 91.2 mg), total purines 119 mg.
- ✓ Carp (hypoxanthine 75 mg), total purines content 103 mg.
- ✓ Salmon roe contains few purines.
- ✓ Sardine (hypoxanthine 87.1 mg), total purine content of 210.4 mg.
- ✓ Tuna (hypoxanthine 129.3 mg), total purine content of 157.4 mg.
- ✓ Rainbow trout (hypoxanthine 99.5 mg), total purine content of 180.9 mg.
- ✓ Mollusks contain a significant amount of purines. Snow crab contains fewer purines 136.4 mg.
- ✓ Fresh mussels have 136 mg of purines, more than canned mussels, which have 62 mg. Canned oysters have 107 mg. Canned salmon contains 88 mg.

The specified amount of purines per 3.53 ounces or 100 grams.

Some supplements, especially DNA/RNA, brewer's yeast, and chlorella contain very high amounts of purine: 21493.6 mg, 2995.7 mg, and 3182.7 mg, respectively. Patients with gout or hyperuricemia should, therefore, avoid taking these supplements. Spirulina contains 1076.8 mg, royal jelly 403.4 mg.

Fatty fish are allowed to reduce the risk of cardiovascular diseases in patients with gout. Some vegetables contain more than 50 mg of purines and are known as purine-rich but do not increase the risk of developing gout.

Products with a low total purine content and products mainly containing adenine and guanine are considered beneficial. These include eggs, dairy products, grains, legumes, vegetables, mushrooms, and soy products. Eggs and dairy products contain virtually no purines.

Milk proteins, such as casein, reduce uric acid concentration in the blood serum by enhancing uric acid removal.

Chapter 4:
Prevention

4.1. Prevention of Gout

The major points of lifestyle interventions are nutritional therapy, restriction of alcohol consumption, and recommendations for physical training. Nutritional therapy suggests an appropriate intake of energy and water (more than two liters) and a reduced intake of dietary purines (less than 400 mg/d) and fructose.

High intake of low-purine foodstuffs, such as dairy products, cereals, beans, vegetables, mushrooms, and soybean products, is strongly recommended. Opt for whole grain products more often to control blood sugar levels.

Make sure to avoid excessive consumption of alcoholic beverages and preferably exclude beer. Excessive alcohol intake leads to more frequent gout recurrences, even when treated with allopurinol.

Consuming foods rich in vitamin C can lower uric acid in the blood serum and reduce the risk of developing gout. It is also beneficial to eat cherries and drink coffee.

Avoid beverages sweetened with high-fructose syrup. It is also recommended to limit the consumption of natural sweetened fruit juices, table sugar, sweetened drinks, desserts, and table salt. Maintaining high hydration levels by consuming ample fluids can help prevent gout flares.

Since the connection between gout and atherosclerosis is well-established, following a low-cholesterol and low-fat diet is prudent.

The daily norm of sugar for men is no more than nine teaspoons, and for women, no more than six teaspoons.

Your taste receptors can adapt to the sweetness level. As you consistently reduce overall sugar intake, you may notice a decreased craving for sweets or find that some products become too sweet.

Examples of medications that can raise uric acid levels:

✓ Diuretics

✓ Low-dose aspirin

✓ Niacin (nicotinic acid)

✓ Testosterone

Weight loss can reduce uric acid levels. However, it is essential to avoid diets that induce ketosis, such as fasting. Experts recommend focusing on long-term and sustainable changes to manage weight.

4.2. Types of Kidney Stones

Patients with gout and kidney stones should avoid foods that contain oxalic acid (spinach, rhubarb, okra, and young beet leaves).

There are four types of kidney stones, but the most common are calcium oxalate and uric acid.

When calcium combines with oxalate in the urine, it forms the most common type of kidney stone: calcium oxalate. Inadequate calcium and fluid intake can contribute to their formation.

Dairy products contain calcium, but they help prevent stone formation. Calcium binds to oxalate before it even reaches the kidneys. People with low calcium intake have a higher risk of kidney stones. Oxalic acid may decrease calcium absorption.

Uric acid is another of the most common types of kidney stones. High purine intake leads to increased formation of monosodium urate, which can form kidney stones.

Eating too much fructose may increase your risk of developing kidney stones.

Drinking enough fluids will help make your urine less concentrated. Most people should drink more than ten glasses of water a day.

Aim to eat more fruits and vegetables to make your urine less acidic. When urine is less acidic, stones are less likely to form. In addition, animal protein may increase the risk of kidney stones.

For people at risk of kidney disease or with a history of kidney stones, it is advisable to limit the consumption of high-oxalate foods.

Foods very high in oxalates

- ✓ Cooked spinach, 1 cup, 1,510 mg
- ✓ Rhubarb, 1 cup, 1,082 mg
- ✓ Okra, 1 cup, 1,014 mg
- ✓ Beet greens, 1 cup, 500 mg

Foods high in oxalates

- ✓ Beets, 1 cup, 152 mg
- ✓ Baked potato with skin, one medium, 97 mg
- ✓ Cornmeal, cooked wheat, 1 cup, 97 mg
- ✓ Soy flour, 1 cup, 94 mg
- ✓ Almonds, 1 ounce (28 g), 122 mg
- ✓ Cocoa powder, 4 teaspoons, 67 mg

When at risk of kidney stone formation:

1. Drink plenty of fluids, 2–3 liters a day.

2. Limit the consumption of high-oxalate foods.

3. Get your calcium from natural sources. Three meals per day   consisting of dairy products can reduce the formation of calcium stones. (1,000–1,200 mg per day.)

4. Discuss calcium supplements with your doctor.

5. Consume a moderate amount of protein.

6. Avoid excessive salt intake.

7. Avoid high doses of vitamin C.

Herbs can be used to prevent inflammatory diseases of the urinary tract.

It is better to select herbal complexes with a doctor. Herbs have indications and contraindications.

4.4. Role of Phytic Acid

Phytic acid binds to part of the minerals. This makes them inaccessible to the body. Phytic acid interferes with iron, zinc, calcium, magnesium, and manganese absorption.

Iron supplements are poorly absorbed with phytic acid products (semolina, beans, peas, etc.). When combined with iron supplements, fresh fruits and vegetables can increase the speed and extent of absorption.

The highest concentration of phytic acid is found in whole grains and legumes. Cooking, soaking overnight in water, fermentation, and marinating can reduce the amount of phytic acid.

Eat vitamin C-rich foods along with phytic acid-containing foods. They significantly counteract the effect of phytic acid.

Rich sources of vitamin C include guava, sweet peppers, kiwi, oranges, grapefruits, strawberries, Brussels sprouts, papaya, broccoli, sweet potatoes, pineapples, cauliflower, and cabbage.

4.5. Natural Products with Anti-Inflammatory Properties

Natural products with anti-inflammatory properties include Andrographis, curcumin (turmeric), resveratrol, quercetin, bromelain, boswellia, black cumin seed oil, and others.

One of the most critical substances found in black pepper is piperine. When combined with curcumin, the bioavailability of curcumin is increased by 2,000%. Indian curry spice contains turmeric and black pepper.

Quercetin is high in plants such as onions, tea, St. John's Wort, and garlic. Its effect is comparable to that of phenylbutazone.

Plants with anti-inflammatory properties include creeping thyme, clove tree (clove spice), bushy sage, medicinal rosemary, marjoram, and wide-leaf lavender. Their effects are comparable to the effects of hydrocortisone.

Pineapples are rich in bromelain, which is an excellent natural anti-inflammatory.

Some individuals are sensitive to a group of foods known as nightshades. For them, consuming nightshades can exacerbate joint pain. Nightshades include potatoes, tomatoes, eggplants, tobacco, and others.

Consuming predominantly plant-based foods is the most effective way to reduce chronic inflammation and joint pain.

Chapter 5:
Physical Activity and Psychological Well-Being

Start with low-intensity workouts, then gradually increase the intensity. Sudden increases in activity can elevate uric acid levels. Exercises with minimal resistance that don't strain the joints can be beneficial. This may include light stretches, flexibility, and coordination exercises. Muscle-toning and stability exercises can help protect the joints. Gentle aerobic activities such as exercise, biking, or walking are recommended.

Regular physical activity, especially between gout attacks, is important to your gout treatment plan. Regular activity can also play a role in weight reduction and help maintain joint mobility.

Everyone has unique needs and limitations, so listening to your body during physical activity is essential.

Living with this condition can be both physically and emotionally draining. It is essential to take proper care of yourself, even when you are not in the midst of an attack.

Warm compresses can improve joint conditions (for prevention). Herbs are available in online stores for dietary supplements and natural products.

COMPRESS WITH CHAMOMILE AND ELDERFLOWER

- ✓ ½ tablespoon chamomile
- ✓ ½ tablespoon elderflower
- ✓ 1 cup boiling water

Simmer on low heat for a couple of minutes, let it cool to an acceptable temperature, then strain. Moisten a cloth, apply it to the joint, cover it with plastic wrap, and wrap it with a black towel to retain warmth.

COMPRESS WITH PLANTAIN AND WORMWOOD

- ✓ ½ tablespoon plantain leaves
- ✓ ½ tablespoon wormwood herb
- ✓ 1 cup boiling water

Simmer for fifteen minutes on low heat, let it cool to an acceptable temperature, then strain. Moisten a cloth, apply it to the joint, cover it with plastic wrap, and wrap it with a black towel to retain warmth.

COMPRESS WITH ST. JOHN'S WORT AND YARROW

- ✓ ½ tablespoon St. John's Wort herb
- ✓ ½ tablespoon yarrow herb
- ✓ 1 cup boiling water

Simmer for fifteen minutes on low heat, let it cool to an acceptable temperature, then strain. Moisten a cloth, apply it to the joint, cover it with plastic wrap, and wrap it with a black towel to retain warmth.

SAFFRON

Saffron is effective against insomnia, stress, and depression and is beneficial for overall immune system strengthening.

- ✓ Brew 1 teaspoon of black tea in one cup of boiling water. In a separate glass, place two saffron threads and pour them with the freshly brewed tea. Steep covered for fifteen minutes. Drink a glass three times a day.

BASIL

Basil slows down the production of cortisol, the stress hormone.

- ✓ Pour 1 cup of slightly cooled boiling water over ½ a tablespoon of freshly chopped basil. Steep covered for twenty minutes. Optionally, add lemon and honey. Drink one glass a day.

Excessive stress can interfere with daily activities, so make sure to prioritize your well-being.

Aromatherapy can be beneficial; choose soothing oils that work for you. They could include cedar, orange, verbena, vanilla, lavender, basil, bergamot, and mint.

Physical exercise, restorative sleep, and a healthy diet can significantly improve mood. The better your mood and outlook, the easier it is to manage gout.

Watch a fun movie or take up a hobby that relaxes you. Meditation, listening to calming music, walks, participating in support groups, and physical exercise can help reduce stress.

Relaxing and slowing down your thoughts through techniques like deep breathing and envisioning images that bring you joy can be beneficial.

Chapter 6:
Breakfast and Snacks

6.1. Oat Flakes with Chia Seeds and Cashews, and Raisins

Prep Time: 5 minutes   Cooking Time: 5 minutes   Servings: 1

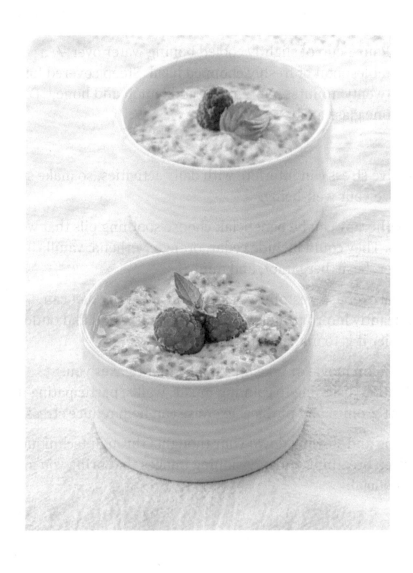

Ingredients

- ½ cup rolled oats
- 1 tablespoon chia seeds
- 2 tablespoons cashews, chopped
- 2 tablespoons raisins
- 1 cup milk (dairy or plant-based)
- 1 teaspoon honey or maple syrup (optional)

Instructions

1. In a small saucepan, add the oats and milk.
2. Turn on the stove to medium heat. Put the saucepan on.
3. Stir the mixture consistently to prevent sticking. Cook for about 3–5 minutes or until the oats are soft.
4. Then, add the chia seeds, chopped cashews, and raisins, stirring to combine.
5. Add honey or maple syrup, to taste.

Nutritional Information (per serving)

Calories: 400 Protein: 13 g Carbohydrates: 58 g

Fat: 14 g Sodium: 50 m

6.2. Oat Flakes with Sesame Seeds, Raisins, and Almonds

Prep Time: 5 minutes   Cooking Time: 5 minutes   Servings: 1

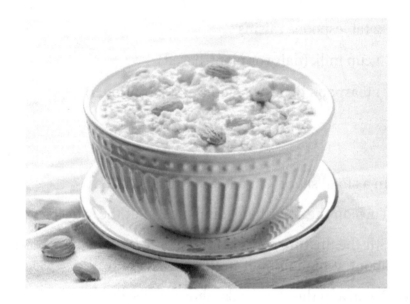

Ingredients

- ½ cup rolled oats
- 1 tablespoon unhulled sesame seeds
- 2 tablespoons raisins
- 1 tablespoon almonds, chopped
- 1 cup milk (dairy or plant-based)
- 1 teaspoon honey or maple syrup (optional)

Instructions

1. In a small saucepan, add the oats and milk.
2. Turn on the stove to medium heat. Put the saucepan on.
3. Stir the mixture consistently to prevent sticking. Cook for about 3–5 minutes or until the oats are soft.
4. Then, add the unhulled sesame seeds, and raisins, and chopped almonds, stirring to combine.
5. Finally, add honey or maple syrup to taste.

Nutritional Information (per serving)

Calories: 450   Protein: 14 g   Carbohydrates: 62 g

Fat: 18 g   Sodium: 60 mg

6.3. Amaranth Porridge with Sesame Seeds, Dried Apricots, and Walnuts

Prep Time: 5 minutes   Cooking Time: 20 minutes   Servings: 1

Ingredients

- ¼ cup amaranth seeds
- 1 cup water
- 1 tablespoon unhulled sesame seeds
- 2 tablespoons chopped dried apricots
- 1 tablespoon chopped walnuts
- A few drops of olive oil
- Honey or maple syrup (optional for sweetness)

Instructions

1. In a small saucepan, combine the rinsed amaranth seeds and water.
2. Bring to a boil. Reduce the heat to low.
3. Cook for about 20 minutes, stirring consistently.
4. Finally, add the unrefined sesame seeds, chopped dried apricots, walnuts, and a few drops of olive oil.
5. If desired, sweeten the porridge with honey or maple syrup, to taste.

Nutritional Information (per serving)

Calories: 350. Protein: 11 g   Carbohydrates: 47 g
Fat: 15 g   Sodium: 80 mg

6.4. Banana and Almond Butter Wrap

Prep Time: 5 minutes   Servings: 1

Ingredients

- 1 whole-grain tortilla or wrap
- 1 tablespoon almond butter
- 1 banana, sliced
- 1 tablespoon chia seeds.
- Drizzle of maple syrup (optional)

Instructions

1. Spread almond butter evenly over the whole-grain tortilla.
2. Place sliced bananas on one side of the tortilla and sprinkle chia seeds on top.
3. Drizzle with maple syrup.

Nutritional Information (per serving)

Calories: 350   Protein: 8 g   Carbohydrates: 50 g

Fat: 14 g   Sodium: 150 mg

6.5. Avocado and Hummus Stuffed Pita Pockets

Prep Time: 10 minutes   Servings: 1

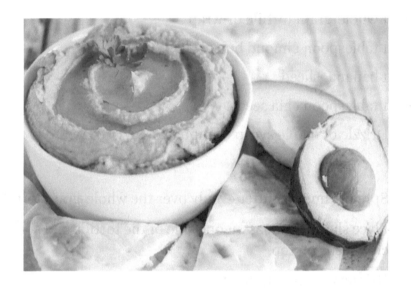

Ingredients

- 1 whole wheat pita bread
- ½ ripe avocado, sliced
- 2 tablespoons hummus
- Cherry tomatoes, halved (optional)
- Fresh cilantro, chopped (optional)
- Salt and pepper, to taste

Instructions

1. If you prefer a warm snack, heat the pita in a pan for about 20–30 seconds on each side.

2. Slice the avocado and halve the cherry tomatoes.

3. Open the pita pockets and spread hummus evenly on the inside surfaces.

4. Place the sliced avocado inside the pita pockets, distributing it evenly.

5. If desired, add halved cherry tomatoes and a sprinkle of fresh cilantro.

6. Season with salt and pepper, to taste.

Nutritional Information (per serving)

Calories: 350 Protein: 8 g Carbohydrates: 38 g

Fat: 19 g Sodium: 350 mg

6.6. Stuffed Mini Bell Peppers

Prep Time: 15 minutes   Servings: 1

Ingredients

- Mini bell peppers
- Hummus
- Cherry tomatoes, halved
- Fresh basil, chopped

Instructions

1. Cut the mini bell peppers in half. Remove the seeds.
2. Fill each pepper half with hummus.
3. Place a halved cherry tomato on top. Sprinkle with fresh basil.

Nutritional Information (per serving)

Calories: 180   Protein: 6 g. Carbohydrates: 25 g

Fat: 8 g. Sodium: 150 mg

Chapter 7:
Legume Dishes

7.1 Vegetarian Meatballs in Tomato Sauce

Prep Time: 20 minutes   Cooking Time: 30–35 minutes

Servings: 4

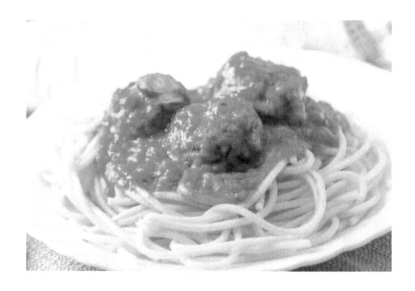

Vegetarian Meatballs

- 1 can (15 oz) of lentils, drained and rinsed
- 1 cup breadcrumbs
- ½ cup grated Parmesan cheese
- ¼ cup finely chopped onion
- 2 cloves garlic, minced
- 1 egg (or a flax egg)*
- 1 teaspoon dried oregano
- Salt and black pepper, to taste
- 2–3 tablespoons olive oil (for frying)
- Cooked pasta or rice

*1 tablespoon of ground flaxseeds with 2 ½ –3 tablespoons of water. Allow the mixture to sit for a few minutes.

Tomato Sauce

- 1 can (28 oz) of crushed tomatoes
- 1 small onion, finely chopped
- 2 cloves garlic, minced
- 1 teaspoon dried basil
- 1 teaspoon dried oregano
- Salt and black pepper, to taste
- 2 tablespoons olive oil

Vegetarian Meatballs

1. Mix the drained lentils and breadcrumbs in a large bowl. Add grated parmesan cheese, chopped onion, minced garlic, and egg (or flax egg). Also, add dried oregano, salt, and black pepper.

2. Mix the ingredients until well combined. If the mixture seems too wet to you, you can add more breadcrumbs. If it's too dry, you can add a little water.

3. Form the mixture into balls the size of meat patties. Line a baking sheet with parchment paper. Place the patties on it.

4. Heat olive oil in a large skillet over high heat. Add the meatballs. Fry them on all sides.

Tomato Sauce

1. Heat olive oil over medium heat. Add the chopped onion and minced garlic. Sauté for about 3–4 minutes.

2. Add crushed tomatoes, basil, oregano, salt, and black pepper. Stir to combine.

3. The sauce should simmer for 10 minutes.

4. Serve over cooked pasta or rice.

Nutritional Information (per serving)

Calories: 300   Protein: 13 g   Carbohydrates: 35 g

Fat: 12 g   Sodium: 760 mg

7.2. Chickpea Pancakes

Prep Time: 15 minutes   Cooking Time: 15 minutes   Servings: 4

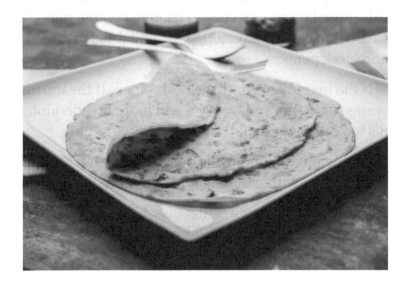

Ingredients

- 1 cup chickpea flour
- 1 ¼ cups water
- 3 tablespoons olive oil
- ½ teaspoon salt
- Fresh cilantro, chopped (optional)
- Optional toppings: cherry tomatoes, olives, herbs, feta cheese

Instructions

1. Whisk together chickpea flour and water in a mixing bowl. Add two tablespoons of olive oil and salt. A smooth batter should result. Let it sit for 15 minutes to allow the flour to absorb the water. Add cilantro.

2. Bake in a pan greased with olive oil.

3. While the pancake is still hot, add toppings such as halved cherry tomatoes, olives, herbs, and crumbled feta cheese.

Nutritional Information (per serving)

Calories: 180   Protein: 6 g   Carbohydrates: 15 g

Fat: 11 g   Sodium: 590 mg

7.3. Adzuki Bean Patties

Prep Time: 14 minutes   Cooking Time: 14 minutes   Servings: 4

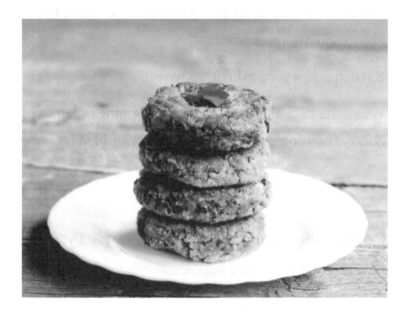

Ingredients

- 1 can (15 oz) adzuki beans, drained and rinsed (you can use any bean)

- 1 cup breadcrumbs

- ¼ cup red onion, finely chopped

- 2 cloves garlic, minced

- ½ teaspoon cumin

- ½ teaspoon paprika

- ½ teaspoon salt

- ¼ teaspoon black pepper

- 2 tablespoons olive oil (for frying)

1. Place the adzuki beans in a large mixing bowl. Mash them with a fork.

2. Add the breadcrumbs and chopped red onion to the bean puree. Also, add the minced garlic, cumin, and paprika. Season, to taste, with salt and black pepper.

3. Mix everything well until you have a uniform mixture. Shape the mixture into patties.

4. Heat the olive oil in a skillet over medium heat. Then, add the patties. Cook for 3–4 minutes on each side or until golden.

5. Serve with a bun and sliced tomatoes.

Nutrition Information (per serving)

Calories: 320 Protein: 11 g Carbohydrates: 50 g

Fat: 8 g Sodium: 620 mg

7.4. Masala with Chickpeas

Prep Time: 15 minutes   Cooking Time: 25 minutes   Servings: 4

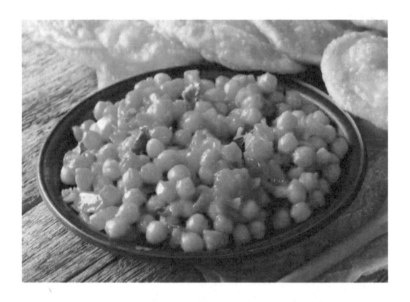

Ingredients

- Two cans (15 ounces each) of chickpeas. The chickpeas should be rinsed and dried.

- 2 tablespoons vegetable oil

- 1 large onion, finely chopped

- 3 cloves garlic, minced

- 1-inch piece of fresh ginger, minced

- 1 teaspoon ground cumin

- 2 teaspoons ground coriander

- ½ teaspoon ground turmeric

- ¼ teaspoon cayenne pepper (adjust to taste)

- 1 can (14 ounces) sliced tomatoes (along with juice)

- 1 cup water

- Salt and black pepper, to taste

- Fresh cilantro leaves for garnish

- Cooked rice or quinoa

1. Heat vegetable oil in a skillet or sauté pan over medium heat. Add the finely chopped onion and sauté 2 minutes. Add the minced garlic and ginger. Continue to sauté for another minute.

2. Add the ground cumin, coriander, turmeric, and cayenne pepper to the skillet. Stir and cook for 2 minutes.

3. Add the chopped tomatoes with their juice to the dish. Stir and cook for 5 minutes.

4. Add the prepared chickpeas to the skillet and stir.

5. Pour in a cup of water and add salt and black pepper, to taste. Bring the mixture to a boil.

6. Cover the skillet and let the Masala simmer over medium heat for 10–15 minutes.

7. Serve over cooked rice or quinoa. Garnish with fresh cilantro.

Nutritional Information (per serving)

Calories: 250   Protein: 10 g   Carbohydrates: 34 g

Fat: 9 g   Sodium: 400 mg

7.5. Eggplant and Lentil

Prep time: 10 minutes   Cooking Time: 35 minutes   Servings: 4

Ingredients

- 1 medium eggplant, diced
- 1 cup green or brown lentils, cooked
- 1 red bell pepper, diced
- 1 zucchini, diced
- 1 onion, chopped
- 3 cloves garlic, minced
- 1 can (14 oz) diced tomatoes
- 2 tablespoons tomato paste
- 1 teaspoon dried thyme
- 1 teaspoon dried oregano
- Salt and pepper, to taste
- 2 tablespoons olive oil
- Cooked rice or quinoa

Instructions

1. In a large skillet, heat the olive oil over medium heat. Add the chopped onion and garlic, and sauté 2 minutes.
2. Add the diced eggplant and cook until it softens and turns golden brown.
3. Add sliced red bell peppers and zucchini. Cook for 2 minutes.
4. Add the cooked lentils, diced tomatoes (with their juice), tomato paste, and hot water. Mix well.
5. Season with dried thyme, oregano, salt, and pepper, and stir.
6. Reduce the heat, cover the pot with a lid, and simmer for 20–25 minutes. The vegetables should become soft.
7. Serve over cooked rice or quinoa.

Nutrition Information (per serving)

Calories: 250   Protein: 11 g   Carbohydrates: 49 g

Fat: 2 g   Sodium: 320 mg

7.6. Casserole with Chickpeas

Prep time: 15 minutes   Cooking Time: 45 minutes   Servings: 4

Ingredients

- Two cans (15 ounces each) of chickpeas
- The chickpeas should be rinsed and dried
- 2 cups of diced butternut
- 2 cups of diced zucchini
- 1 red bell pepper, diced
- 1 red onion, diced
- 2 cloves of garlic, minced
- 1 can (14.5 oz) of diced tomatoes (with juice)
- ½ cup vegetable broth or water
- 1 teaspoon dried thyme
- 1 teaspoon dried rosemary
- 1 teaspoon paprika
- Salt and black pepper, to taste
- 2 tablespoons olive oil
- 1 cup shredded mozzarella cheese (optional)

1. Take a large oven-safe casserole. Heat the olive oil over medium heat.

2. Add the chopped onion and garlic, and sauté 2 minutes.

3. Add the dish's diced butternut, zucchini, and red bell pepper. Sauté for another 5 minutes or until the vegetables start to soften.

4. Heat oven to 375°F (190°C).

5. Add the chickpeas, dried thyme, rosemary, and paprika to the dish, vegetable broth, or water. Season to taste with salt and black pepper to taste. Cook for an additional 2 minutes.

6. Pour the diced tomatoes and their juice into the broth. Stir and add cheese.

7. Cover the casserole with a lid or foil. Place in the oven. Bake for 30–35 minutes. The vegetables should become soft.

Nutritional Information (per serving)

Calories: 340   Protein: 11 g   Carbohydrates: 51 g

Fat: 11 g   Sodium: 860 mg

7.7. Lentil Dal

Prep Time: 15 minutes   Cooking Time: 30–40 minutes
Servings: 4

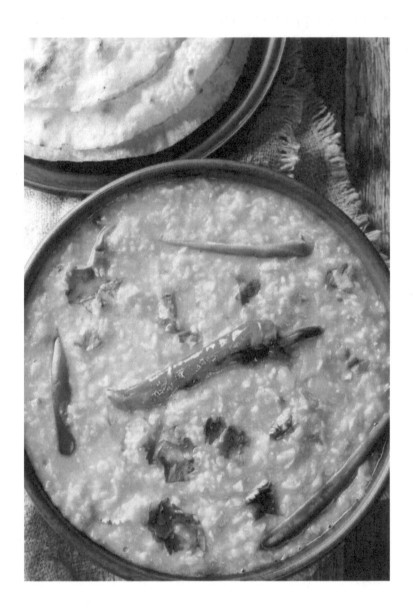

Ingredients

- 1 cup dry lentils (red or yellow lentils work well)
- 4 cups water
- 2 tablespoons olive oil or vegetable oil
- 1 large onion, finely chopped
- 3 cloves garlic, minced
- 1 tablespoon fresh ginger, grated
- 1 teaspoon curry powder
- ¼ teaspoon turmeric
- A pinch of cayenne pepper
- 1 can (14 oz) diced tomatoes
- 1 can (14 oz) coconut milk
- Salt and pepper, to taste
- Fresh cilantro, chopped (for garnish)
- Cooked rice

Instructions

1. Rinse the lentils under cold water.
2. In a large pot, combine the lentils and water. Bring to a boil. Reduce heat to low, cover, and simmer for about 20–25 minutes. The lentils should become soft.
3. Heat the oil over medium heat in a separate skillet. Add chopped onions and sauté 2 minutes.
4. Add grated ginger. Sauté for an additional 1 minute.
5. Add curry powder, cayenne pepper, and turmeric. Cook for 1–2 minutes.
6. Add the diced tomatoes with their juice to the spice mixture. Cook for another 3 minutes.

7. Pour in coconut milk. Season with salt and pepper. The mixture should simmer for 10 minutes.

8. Once the lentils are cooked, add lentils. Stir well and let the dal simmer for 5 minutes.

9. Adjust salt and pepper, to taste.

10. Serve the dal over cooked rice, garnished with chopped fresh cilantro.

Nutritional Information (per serving)

Calories: 380. Protein: 14 g Carbohydrates: 45 g

Fat: 17 g Sodium: 750 mg

Chapter 8:
Vegetable Dishes

8.1. Pumpkin Risotto

Prep Time: 15 minutes   Cooking Time: 30–35 minutes
Servings: 4

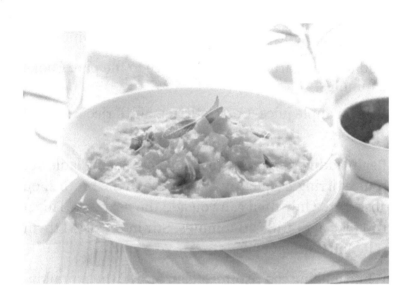

Ingredients

- 2 cups Arborio rice
- 1 small pumpkin (2 pounds), peeled, seeded, and diced into small cubes
- 1 onion, finely chopped
- 2 cloves of garlic, minced
- 1 cup apple juice
- 4 cups vegetable broth
- 3 tablespoons olive oil

- ½ cup Parmesan cheese

- 1 teaspoon dried thyme

- Salt and black pepper, to taste

Instructions

1. Heat vegetable broth in a large saucepan. Keep it warm but not boiling.

2. Take a large, deep frying pan or saucepan. Heat olive oil over medium heat. Add onion and sauté 2 minutes.

3. Add minced garlic and Arborio rice to the pan. Cook for 2 minutes.

4. Pour in apple juice. Cook, stirring, until rice is almost absorbed.

5. Begin adding the warm vegetable broth, one ladle at a time, stirring frequently. Each ladle of the broth should be absorbed. Only then can you add the next one. This process will take about 18–20 minutes. Stir in the dried thyme, salt, and black pepper.

6. While making the risotto, steam or boil the pumpkin cubes in a separate pan until they are tender. This will take about 10–12 minutes.

7. Once the pumpkin is tender, mash half with a fork and leave the other half in cubes for texture.

8. Remove it from the heat when the risotto is creamy and the rice is cooked.

9. Stir in the mashed pumpkin-grated Parmesan cheese. Mix until well combined, then add pumpkin cubes.

Nutritional Information (per serving)

Calories: 390   Protein: 9 g   Carbohydrates: 72 g

Fat: 10 g   Sodium: 1 mg

8.2. Stuffed Bell Peppers

Prep Time: 20 minutes   Cooking Time: 30–35 minutes
Servings: 4

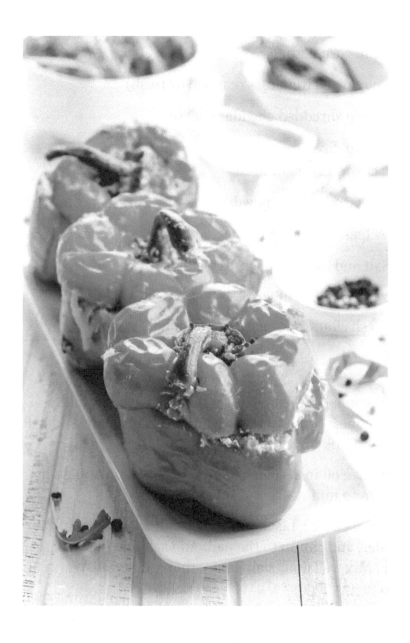

Ingredients

- 4 large bell peppers (red, green, or yellow)
- 1 cup cooked rice (white or brown)
- 1 can (14 oz) black beans, drained and rinsed
- 1 cup corn kernels
- 1 cup diced tomatoes (canned or fresh)
- ½ cup shredded cheddar cheese
- ½ cup diced red onion
- 2 cloves garlic, minced
- ¼ teaspoon chili powder
- ½ teaspoon cumin
- Salt and black pepper, to taste
- 2 tablespoons olive oil
- Fresh cilantro for garnish (optional)

Instructions

1. Cut the tops off the bell peppers. Remove seeds and membranes. Bring water to a boil in a saucepan. Add bell pepper. Cook for 3 minutes.

2. Heat olive oil in a saucepan. Add diced onion and garlic. Cook for 2 minutes.

3. Add cooked rice, black beans, corn, diced tomatoes, chili powder, and cumin to the pan. Add salt and black pepper, to taste. Mix well and cook for another 3 minutes. Warm up the oven to 375°F (190°C).

4. Add ½ cup shredded cheddar cheese.

5. Gently stuff each bell pepper with the mixture from the skillet.

6. Place the stuffed peppers in a baking dish. Sprinkle with grated cheddar cheese.

7. Bake in the oven for 25 minutes or until the peppers are tender.

8. Garnish with fresh cilantro if desired.

Nutritional Information (per serving)

Calories: 360   Protein: 14 g   Carbohydrates: 61 g

Fat: 10 g   Sodium: 710 mg

8.3. Caprese Pasta

Prep Time: 15 minutes Cooking Time: 10–15 minutes Servings: 4

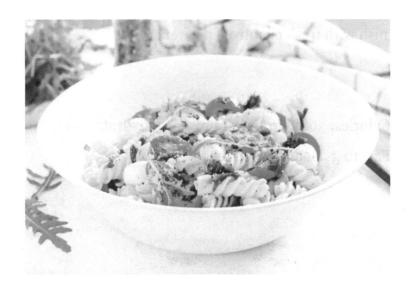

Ingredients

- 12 ounces (about 340 g) of pasta
- 4 large tomatoes, ripe and diced
- 1 cup fresh mozzarella cheese, diced
- ¼ cup fresh basil leaves, chopped
- 2–3 cloves of garlic, minced
- ¼ cup extra-virgin olive oil
- ¼ teaspoon lemon juice
- Salt and black pepper, to taste
- Grated Parmesan cheese (optional for serving)

Instructions

1. Prepare pasta as directed on the package.

2. Combine diced tomatoes and fresh mozzarella in a bowl. Add chopped basil and minced garlic.

3. Place extra virgin olive oil and lemon juice in a small bowl. Salt and black pepper, to taste.

4. Pour the prepared dressing over the tomato and mozzarella mixture. Mix well. Let it sit for about 5 minutes.

5. Transfer the cooked pasta to a bowl with the tomato and mozzarella mixture. Mix well. Serve with grated Parmesan cheese.

Nutritional Information (per serving)

Calories: 450 Protein: 15 g Carbohydrates: 50 g

Fat: 22 g Sodium: 260 mg

8.4. Spanish Vegetable Stew

Prep Time: 15–20 minutes   Cooking Time: 30–35 minutes
Servings: 4

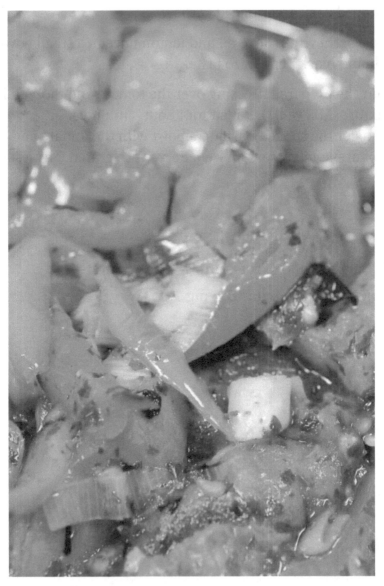

Ingredients

- 2 tablespoons olive oil

- 1 onion, finely chopped

- 1 red bell pepper, diced

- 1 yellow bell pepper, diced

- 1 small zucchini, diced

- 1 small eggplant, diced

- 3 cloves garlic, minced

- 1 can (14 oz) diced tomatoes

- 1 teaspoon smoked paprika

- ½ teaspoon cumin

- Salt and black pepper, to taste

Instructions

1. In a large frying pan, heat the olive oil over medium heat.

2. Add the finely chopped onion and sauté for 3 minutes.

3. Add chopped garlic. Sauté for 1 minute.

4. Stir in the diced zucchini and eggplant. Cook for another 5 minutes. The vegetables should become soft.

5. Add chopped red and yellow bell peppers to the pan. Sauté for about 5 minutes.

6. Pour in the can of diced tomatoes with their juices. Add cumin, salt, and black pepper. Stir to combine.

7. Cover the skillet and let it simmer for 15 minutes over medium heat.

8. Add smoked paprika.

Nutritional Information (per serving)

Calories: 110   Protein: 2 g   Carbohydrates: 19 g

Fat: 4 g   Sodium: 330 mg

8.5. Vegetable Stew

Prep Time: 15 minutes   Cooking Time: 30 minutes   Servings: 4

Ingredients

- 2 tablespoons olive oil
- 1 onion, chopped
- 2 cloves garlic, minced
- 1 carrot, peeled and diced
- 2 potatoes, peeled and diced
- 1 small bell pepper, diced
- 1 small zucchini, diced
- 1 can (15 oz) diced tomatoes
- 3 cups vegetable broth or water
- ½ cup green beans peeled and cut into small pieces
- ½ cup corn kernels
- ½ cup fresh or frozen peas
- ¼ teaspoon paprika
- A pinch of hot peppers
- Salt and black pepper, to taste

Instructions

1. Heat olive oil in a saucepan.

2. Add the chopped onion and minced garlic. Sauté for 2 minutes.

3. Add chopped carrots and potatoes to the pan. Sauté for 5 minutes, stirring.

4. Add chopped bell peppers, zucchini, and a can of chopped tomatoes with their juice. Pour in vegetable broth or water. Add spices.

5. Add the green beans, corn kernels, and peas to the stew. Season with salt, black pepper, hot peppers, and paprika.

6. Continue to simmer for another 20 minutes.

7. Once all the vegetables are cooked, remove the pot from the heat.

Nutritional Information (per serving)

Calories: 230   Protein: 7 g   Carbohydrates: 45 g

Fat: 4 g   Sodium: 780 mg

Chapter 9:
Bread Spread

9.1. Hummus with Sesame Paste (Tahini)

Prep Time: 10 minutes   Servings: 4

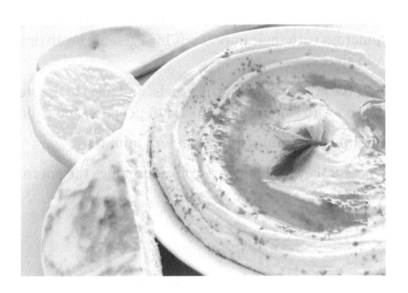

Ingredients

- Two cans (15 ounces each) of chickpeas. The water must be drained and washed.

- ½ cup tahini (sesame paste)

- ¼ cup extra-virgin olive oil, plus more for serving

- 2 cloves garlic, minced

- 1 tablespoon lemon juice

- Salt, to taste

- Water (as needed for consistency)

- ½ teaspoon smoked paprika for garnish

If using canned chickpeas, drain and rinse them under cold water.

1. Combine chickpeas, tahini, olive oil, minced garlic, and lemon juice in a food processor.

2. Mix all ingredients until smooth texture. If the mixture appears too thick, gradually incorporate water, one tablespoon at a time, until you reach the desired consistency.

3. Add salt, to taste.

4. Transfer the hummus to a serving bowl. Create a well in the center and drizzle with olive oil. Sprinkle with smoked paprika.

Nutritional Information (per serving)

Calories: 300   Protein: 10 g   Carbohydrates: 25 g

Fat: 18 g   Sodium: 200 mg

9.2. Avocado and Herb Spread

Prep Time: 10 minutes   Servings: 4

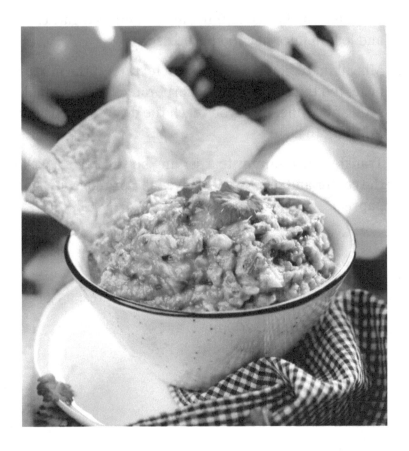

Ingredients

- 2 ripe avocados
- ½ teaspoon fresh lemon juice
- 2 cloves garlic, minced
- ¼ cup fresh basil, chopped
- ¼ cup fresh chives, chopped
- 2–3 tablespoons extra-virgin olive oil
- Red pepper flakes (optional, for a hint of spice)
- Salt and black pepper, to taste

Instructions

1. Cut the ripe avocado in half. Place the pulp in a bowl.
2. Add the fresh lemon juice to the avocados. Mash the avocado with a fork until smooth.
3. Add the minced garlic, fresh basil, and chopped chives.
4. Add salt and black pepper, to taste. You can also add red pepper flakes.
5. Add 2–3 tablespoons of extra-virgin olive oil into the mixture and stir until well combined.

Nutritional Information (per serving)

Calories: 150   Protein: 2 g   Carbohydrates: 8 g

Fat: 14 g   Sodium: 300 mg

9.3. Olive Tapenade Spread

Prep Time: 10 minutes   Servings: 4

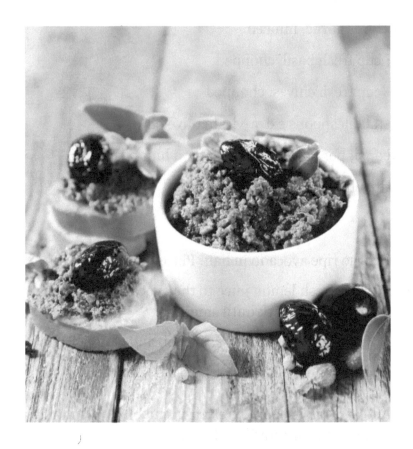

Ingredients

- 1 cup pitted black olives
- ½ cup pitted green olives
- 2 cloves garlic, minced
- ½ teaspoon fresh lemon juice
- 2 tablespoons extra-virgin olive oil
- Fresh basil for garnish (optional)

Instructions

1. Grind black olives, green olives, and minced garlic in a food processor.
2. Add fresh lemon juice.
3. Add extra virgin olive oil.
4. Garnish with fresh basil.

Nutritional Information (per serving)

Calories: 100. Protein: 0 g   Carbohydrates: 2 g

Fat: 11 g   Sodium: 780 mg

9.4. Sun-Dried Tomato Spread

Prep Time: 10 minutes   Servings: 4

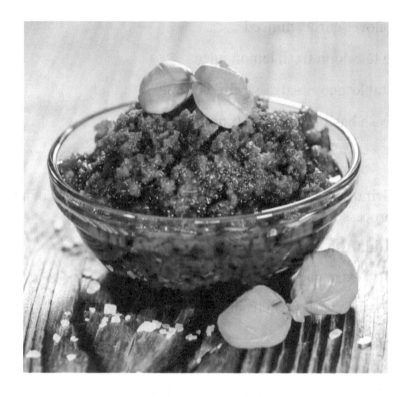

Ingredients

- 1 cup sun-dried tomatoes (not in oil)
- ½ cup raw cashews
- 2 cloves garlic, minced
- 2 tablespoons extra-virgin olive oil
- ½ teaspoon fresh lemon juice
- ½ teaspoon dried basil
- ¼ teaspoon dried oregano
- Salt and black pepper, to taste

Instructions

1. If the cashews are not pre-soaked, you can do a quick soak by placing them in a bowl, pouring boiling water over them, and letting them sit for 10 minutes, then drain.

2. Combine sun-dried tomatoes, cashews, garlic, extra virgin olive oil, fresh lemon juice, dried basil, dried oregano, salt, and black pepper in a food processor.

Nutritional Information (per serving)

Calories: 170   Protein: 5 g   Carbohydrates: 14 g

Fat: 11 g   Sodium: 230 mg

9.5. Spicy pumpkin spread

Prep Time: 10 minutes

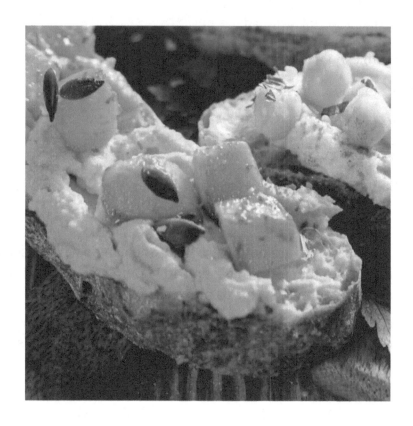

Ingredients

- 1 cup canned pumpkin puree (unsweetened)
- 4 ounces cream cheese, softened
- 2 cloves garlic, minced
- 1 tablespoon olive oil
- 1 teaspoon ground cumin
- ½ teaspoon smoked paprika
- A pinch of cayenne pepper (adjust to taste)
- Salt, to taste
- Chopped fresh cilantro for garnish (optional)

Instructions

1. In a medium bowl, combine the canned pumpkin puree, cream cheese, garlic, olive oil, cumin, smoked paprika, and cayenne pepper.
2. Add salt to taste.
3. Mix until well combined.
4. Garnish with fresh cilantro.

Nutritional Information (per serving)

Calories: 90   Protein: 2 g   Carbohydrates: 5 g

Fat: 7 g   Sodium: 160 mg

9.6. Bean Spread and Fried Vegetable

Prep Time: 20 minutes   Cooking Time: 15 minutes   Servings: 4

Ingredients

Bean Spread

- 1 can (15 oz) of white beans, drained and rinsed
- 2 cloves garlic, minced
- 2 tablespoons extra-virgin olive oil
- ½ teaspoon fresh lemon juice
- ¼ teaspoon ground cumin
- Salt and black pepper, to taste

Fried Vegetables

- 1 zucchini, diced
- 1 red bell pepper, diced
- 1 small eggplant, diced
- 2 tablespoons olive oil
- ½ teaspoon paprika or smoked paprika
- Salt and black pepper, to taste

Bean Spread

Combine the white beans, minced garlic, extra-virgin olive oil, fresh lemon juice, ground cumin, salt, and black pepper in a food processor.

Fried Vegetables

1. Heat two tablespoons of olive oil in a skillet over medium-high heat.

2. Add the diced zucchini, red bell pepper, and eggplant to the skillet.

3. Add salt, paprika, and black pepper to vegetables, to taste.

4. Sauté the vegetables for about 10–15 minutes, stirring occasionally, until they are tender.

Nutritional Information (per serving)

Calories: 180   Protein: 5 g   Carbohydrates: 22 g

Fat: 8 g   Sodium: 230 mg

9.7. White Bean and Roasted Red Bell Pepper Bread Spread

Prep Time: 10 minutes. Servings: 4

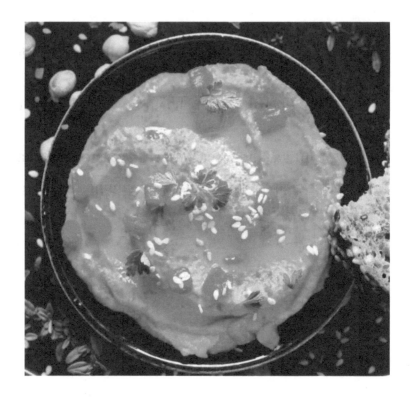

Ingredients

- 1 can (15 oz) white beans, drained and rinsed
- 1 cup roasted red bell pepper from a jar, drained and patted dry
- 2 cloves garlic, minced
- 2 tablespoons fresh basil, chopped
- ½ teaspoon lemon juice
- Salt and black pepper, to taste

Instructions

Combine the white beans, bell peppers, minced garlic, fresh basil, lemon juice, salt, and black pepper in a food processor.

Nutritional Information (per serving)

Calories: 150. Protein: 6 g   Carbohydrates: 28 g

Fat: 1 g   Sodium: 350 mg

9.8. Spread with Red Bell Pepper and Walnut

Prep Time: 20 minutes   Servings: 4

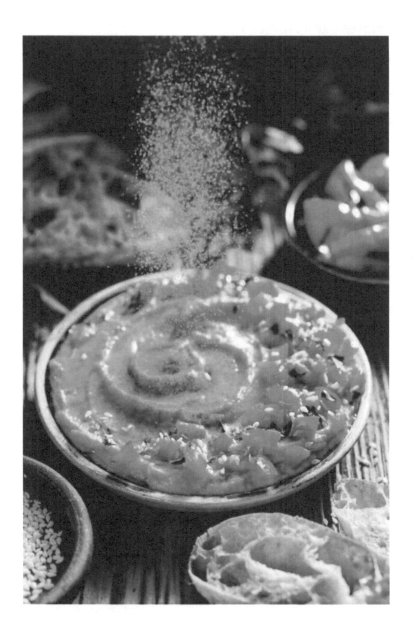

- 2 large red bell peppers, chopped

- 1 cup walnuts

- 2 cloves garlic, minced

- ½ teaspoon fresh lemon juice

- 2 tablespoons extra-virgin olive oil

- Salt and black pepper, to taste

Instructions

1. Fry bell peppers in olive oil.

2. Combine the roasted red peppers, walnuts, minced garlic, fresh lemon juice, extra-virgin olive oil, salt, and black pepper in a food processor.

Nutritional Information (per serving)

Calories: 200   Protein: 4 g   Carbohydrates: 6 g

Fat: 18 g   Sodium: 95 mg

Chapter 10:
Tofu Dishes

10.1. Tofu and Vegetable Curry

Prep Time: 15 minutes   Cooking Time: 20 minutes   Servings: 4

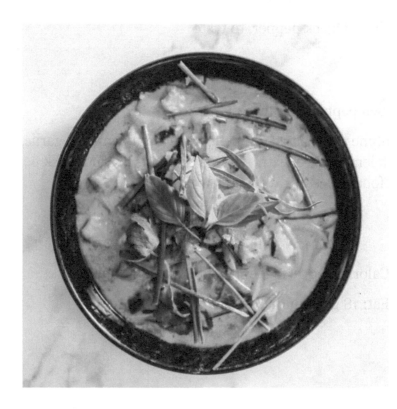

Ingredients

- 14 oz (400 g) extra-firm tofu, cubed
- 1 can (14 oz) coconut milk
- 1 cup bell peppers and peas
- 1 medium onion
- 4 cloves garlic
- Small piece of ginger
- 1 tablespoon red curry paste
- 1 tablespoon vegetable oil
- ½ teaspoon coconut sugar (or to taste)
- Salt, to taste
- Cooked rice for serving

Instructions

1. Heat vegetable oil in a frying pan over medium-high heat.
2. Add diced tofu. Stir the fry for 5 minutes until golden brown. Remove from the skillet and set aside.
3. Add onions and garlic to the pan. Sauté for 2 minutes. Add ginger and red curry paste. Pour in the coconut milk. Add sugar. Cook for 1 minute, stirring constantly. Add the mixed vegetables and cook for 12 minutes.
4. Return the cooked tofu to the pan. Add salt and stir.
5. Serve the tofu and vegetable curry over cooked rice.

Nutritional Information (per serving)

Calories: 280 Protein: 11 g Carbohydrates: 14 g

Fat: 21 g Sodium: 480 mg

10.2. Tofu Stir-Fry

Prep Time: 15 minutes   Cooking Time: 15 minutes   Servings: 4

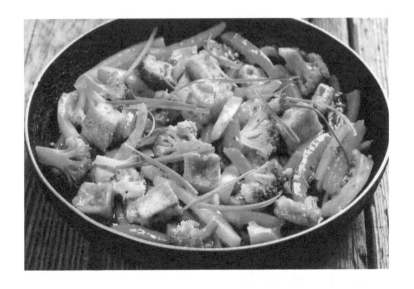

Ingredients

- 14 oz (400 g) firm tofu, cubed

- Two cups of mixed vegetables (bell peppers, broccoli, carrots, peas, etc.). Everything is cut into slices.

- 1 tablespoon low-sodium soy sauce

- 1 tablespoons maple syrup or agave nectar

- 2 cloves garlic, minced

- ½ tablespoon ginger, minced

- 2 tablespoons vegetable oil

- Cooked rice for serving

Instructions

1. Take a small bowl to prepare the sauce. Mix soy sauce and maple syrup (or agave nectar). Add chopped garlic and ginger.

2. Pour one tablespoon of vegetable oil into the pan. Reheat well.

3. Add diced tofu. Fry, stirring, about 5 minutes, until golden brown. Remove from the skillet and set aside.

4. Pour one tablespoon of vegetable oil into the pan. Reheat well. Add chopped vegetables. Fry, stirring everything, for about 7 minutes until it is done.

5. Return the cooked tofu to the pan. Pour the sauce over the tofu and vegetables. Mix well.

6. Cook for an additional 2 minutes.

7. Serve with cooked rice.

Nutritional Information (per serving)

Calories: 250   Protein: 12 g   Carbohydrates: 23 g

Fat: 12 g   Sodium: 750 mg

10.3. Crumbled Tofu

Prep Time: 10 minutes   Cooking Time: 15 minutes   Servings: 4

Ingredients

- 14 oz (400 g) extra-firm tofu, crumbled
- ½ red bell pepper, diced
- ½ green bell pepper, diced
- ½ onion, diced
- 2 cloves garlic, minced
- ¼ teaspoon turmeric (for color)
- ¼ teaspoon cumin
- 1 tablespoon olive oil
- Salt and black pepper, to taste

Instructions

1. Heat the olive oil in a large skillet over medium heat.
2. Add the diced onions and sauté for 3 minutes.
3. Add chopped red and green bell peppers. Add chopped garlic. Sauté for an additional 3 minutes.
4. Add the crumbled tofu, turmeric, cumin, salt, and black pepper. Cook, stirring occasionally, for about 10 minutes.
5. Serve the tofu with toast.

Nutritional Information (per serving)

Calories: 140Protein: 14 g Carbohydrates: 7 g

Fat: 7 g Sodium: 290 mg

This page is for
YOUR NOTES

Chapter 11:
Mushroom Dishes

11.1. Stuffed Mushrooms

Prep Time: 15 minutes   Cooking Time: 20 minutes   Servings: 4

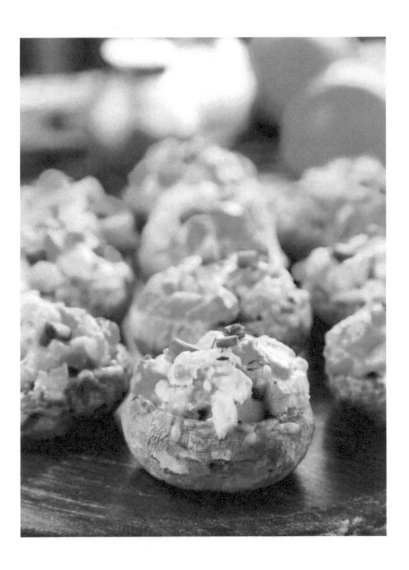

Ingredients

- 16 large white button mushrooms (champignons)
- 2 tablespoons olive oil
- 1 small onion, finely chopped
- 1 tomato chopped
- 2 cloves garlic, minced
- ½ cup breadcrumbs
- ½ cup grated Parmesan cheese
- ¼ cup green onions
- Salt and pepper, to taste

Instructions

1. Clean the mushrooms. First, place the mushroom caps on a baking sheet.
2. Finely chop the mushroom stems.
3. Turn the frying pan over medium heat. Heat the olive oil in it. Add chopped onions. Sauté onions until they turn golden.
4. Add chopped mushroom stems to the pan. Cook for another 3–4 minutes. Warm up your oven to 375°F (190°C).
5. Combine the sautéed mushroom mixture with breadcrumbs, grated Parmesan, tomato, green onions, minced garlic, salt, and pepper. Mix well.
6. Fill each mushroom cap with the prepared filling. Each cap should be pressed down slightly.
7. Bake stuffed mushrooms for 20–25 minutes.

Nutritional Information (per serving)

Calories: 150   Protein: 6 g   Carbohydrates: 14 g

Fat: 9 g   Sodium: 250 mg

11.2. Garlic Mushroom Pasta

Prep Time: 15 minutes   Cooking Time: 15 minutes   Servings: 4

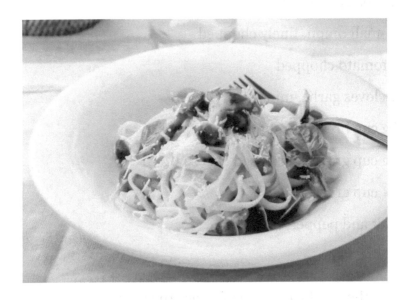

Ingredients

- 12 oz (340 g) pasta
- 1 lb (450 g) mushrooms, cleaned and sliced
- 3 tablespoons olive oil
- 4 cloves garlic, minced
- Salt and black pepper, to taste
- Grated Parmesan cheese (for serving)

Instructions

1. Cook the pasta. Drain and set aside.
2. Turn the frying pan over medium heat. Heat the olive oil in it.
3. Add chopped mushrooms to the pan. Fry them until golden brown.
4. Add minced garlic to the mushrooms and sauté for another 2 minutes.
5. Season with salt and black pepper, to taste.
6. Add cooked pasta to the pan. Mix everything.
7. Serve the pasta hot, topped with grated Parmesan cheese.

Nutritional Information (per serving)

Calories: 400   Protein: 10 g   Carbohydrates: 60 g

Fat: 14 g   Sodium: 80 mg

11.3. Eringi Mushroom and Onion Stir-Fry

Prep Time: 10 minutes   Cooking Time: 15 minutes   Servings: 4

Ingredients

- 4 large eringi mushrooms, cleaned and sliced
- 2 large onions, thinly sliced
- 3 tablespoons olive oil
- Salt and pepper, to taste

Instructions

1. Heat the olive oil in a large skillet.
2. Add sliced onions to the pan. Stir-fry for 4 minutes.
3. Add sliced eringi mushrooms. Cook for 11 minutes.
4. Add salt and pepper, to taste.

Nutritional Information (per serving)

Calories: 180. Protein: 5 g. Carbohydrates: 15 g

Fat: 12 g   Sodium: 10 mg

Chapter 12:
Tarts

12.1. Mediterranean Vegetable Tart

Prep Time: 20 minutes   Cooking Time: 25 minutes. Servings: 4

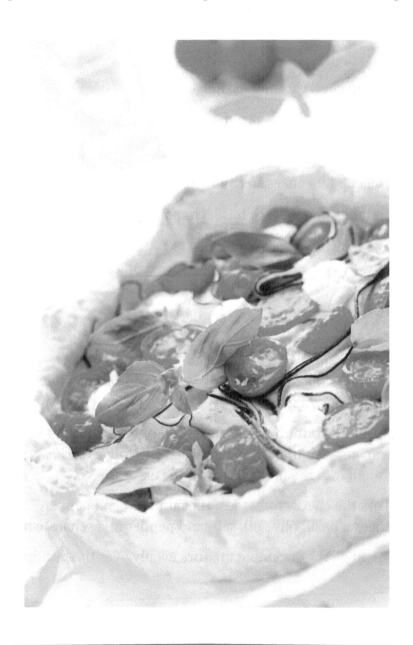

Ingredients

Crust

- 1 ½ cups all-purpose flour
- ¼ cup olive oil
- ¼ cup cold water
- ½ teaspoon salt

Filling

- 1 cup cherry tomatoes, halved
- 1 zucchini, thinly sliced
- 1 red bell pepper, thinly sliced
- ½ cup feta cheese, crumbled
- 2 tablespoons fresh basil, chopped
- 3 tablespoons olive oil
- Salt and pepper, to taste

Instructions

1. Heat oven to 375°F (190°C).
2. Combine the flour, olive oil, water, and salt in a bowl. Mix until a dough forms.
3. Sprinkle flour on the surface. Roll out the dough. Then, transfer it to the tart pan greased with olive oil. Place the dough into the mold. Trim off the excess.
4. Toss the cherry tomatoes, zucchini, red bell pepper, feta cheese, basil, olive oil, salt, and pepper in a separate bowl.
5. Arrange the vegetable mixture evenly over the tart crust.

6. Bake in the oven for about 25 minutes or until the crust is golden and the vegetables are tender.

7. Allow the tart to cool for a few minutes before slicing and serving.

Nutritional Information (per serving)

Calories: 320   Protein: 8 g   Carbohydrates: 30 g

Fat: 20 g   Sodium: 420 mg

12.2. Tomato and Goat Cheese Tart

Prep Time: 20 minutes   Cooking Time: 30 minutes   Servings: 4

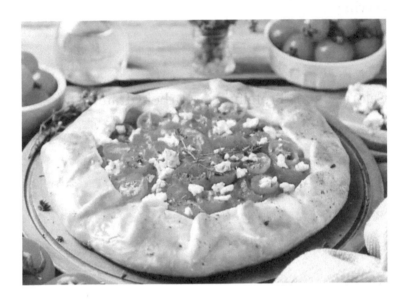

Ingredients

Crust

- 1 ¼ cups all-purpose flour
- ¼ cup olive oil
- ¼ cup cold water
- ½ teaspoon salt

Filling

- 4 medium tomatoes, sliced
- ½ cup goat cheese, crumbled
- 1 tablespoons fresh thyme, chopped
- 2 tablespoons olive oil
- Salt and pepper, to taste

Instructions

1. Heat oven to 375°F (190°C).
2. Combine the flour, olive oil, water, and salt in a bowl. Mix until a dough forms.
3. Dust the surface with flour. Roll out the dough and transfer to a baking sheet greased with olive oil.
4. Place the tomato slices in the center of the dough. It is necessary to leave space at the edges.
5. Sprinkle goat cheese and thyme over the tomatoes. Drizzle with olive oil, and season with salt and pepper.
6. Fold the edges of the dough over the tomatoes.
7. Bake in the oven for about 30 minutes or until the crust is golden and the tomatoes are tender.
8. Allow to cool for a few minutes before slicing and serving.

Nutritional Information (per serving)

Calories: 280   Protein: 7 g. Carbohydrates: 20 g

Fat: 19 g   Sodium: 230 mg

12.3. Roasted Vegetable and Goat Cheese Galette

Prep Time: 20 minutes   Cooking Time: 30 minutes   Servings: 4

Ingredients

Crust

- 1 ¼ cups all-purpose flour
- ¼ cup olive oil
- ¼ cup cold water
- ½ teaspoon salt

Filling

- 1 zucchini, thinly sliced
- 1 yellow bell pepper, thinly sliced
- 1 red onion, thinly sliced
- 2 tablespoons olive oil
- 4 ounces goat cheese, crumbled
- Salt and pepper, to taste
- 2 tablespoons fresh thyme leaves

Instructions

1. Heat oven to 375°F (190°C).
2. Combine the flour, olive oil, water, and salt in a bowl. Mix until a dough forms.
3. Dust the surface with flour. Roll out the dough and transfer to a baking sheet greased with olive oil.

4. In a bowl, toss together the sliced zucchini, yellow bell pepper, red onion, olive oil, salt, and pepper.

5. Place the vegetable mixture in the center of the rolled-out dough. Leaving space around the edges.

6. Crumble the goat cheese over the vegetables. Sprinkle thyme over everything. Bake in the oven for about 30 minutes or until the crust is golden and the vegetables are tender.

7. Allow to cool for a few minutes before slicing and serving.

Nutritional Information (per serving)

Calories: 320   Protein: 8 g   Carbohydrates: 22 g

Fat: 23 g   Sodium: 550 mg

12.4. Flatbreads without Yeast

Prep Time: 10–15 minutes   Cooking Time: 15–20 minutes

Servings: 4

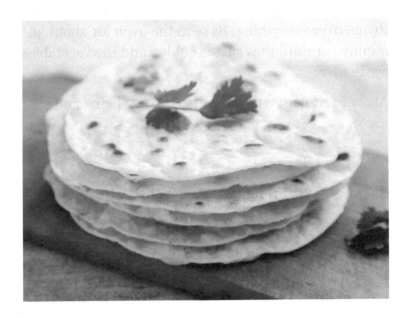

Ingredients

- 2 cups all-purpose flour
- 1 teaspoon baking powder
- ⅔ cup water
- ½ teaspoon salt

Instructions

1. In a bowl, combine all-purpose flour and baking powder. Add salt.

2. Gently add water while stirring the mixture lightly. Continue adding water. The dough should become smooth. You may not need the full ⅔ cup of water.

3. Knead the dough on a lightly floured surface for about 4–5 minutes. It should become smooth and elastic.

4. Divide the dough into four equal parts. Roll each part into a ball.

5. Roll out each ball of dough into a thin, flat round. Brush one side of the flatbread with oil.

6. Place one of the flatbreads in the hot, dry, large skillet. Cook for 2 minutes on each side or until it puffs up and has golden brown spots.

7. Remove the cake from the pan. Cover it with a paper towel or clean cloth.

Nutritional Information (per serving)

Calories: 200 Protein: 4 g Carbohydrates: 40 g

Fat: 1 g Sodium: 295 mg

Chapter 13:
Cookies and Cakes

13.1. Olive Oil and Lemon Cookies

Prep Time: 15 minutes   Cooking Time: 25 minutes   Servings: 4

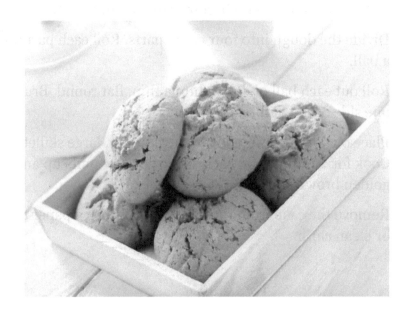

- ½ cup olive oil
- ¾ cup granulated sugar
- 1 large egg
- 1 teaspoon lemon zest
- 1 tablespoon fresh lemon juice
- 1 ¾ cups all-purpose flour
- ½ teaspoon baking powder
- A pinch of salt
- Powdered sugar for dusting (optional)

Instructions

1. Heat oven to 350°F (180°C). Line a baking sheet with parchment paper.
2. Combine olive oil and granulated sugar in a large bowl. Add the egg, zest, and lemon juice.
3. In another bowl, whisk flour, baking powder, and salt.
4. Add dry ingredients to wet ingredients. Mix everything thoroughly.
5. Take a tablespoon and place the dough on the baking sheet one at a time.
6. Bake for 25 minutes.
7. If desired, you can sprinkle the cooled cookies with powdered sugar.

Nutritional Information (per serving)

Calories: 180   Protein: 2 g   Carbohydrates: 24 g

Total Fat: 9 g   Sodium: 70 mg

13.2. Lemon Ricotta Olive Oil Cookies

Prep Time: 15 minutes   Cooking Time: 25 minutes   Servings: 4

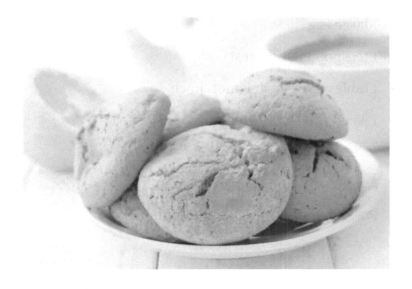

Ingredients

- 1 cup all-purpose flour
- ½ cup nut flour (or additional all-purpose flour)
- ½ teaspoon baking powder
- ½ cup olive oil
- ¾ cup granulated sugar
- 1 large egg
- 1 teaspoon vanilla extract
- Zest of 1 lemon
- 2 tablespoons fresh lemon juice
- ½ cup ricotta cheese
- A pinch of salt

Instructions

1. Heat oven to 350°F (180 °C). Line a baking sheet with parchment paper.

2. Combine all-purpose flour, nut flour, salt, and baking powder in a medium bowl.

3. Whisk together the olive oil, granulated sugar, egg, vanilla extract, lemon zest, and lemon juice in another bowl.

4. Add ricotta cheese to the wet ingredients.

5. Add dry ingredients to wet ingredients. Mix everything thoroughly.

6. Take a tablespoon and place the dough on the baking sheet one at a time.

7. Bake for 25 minutes.

Nutritional Information (per serving)

Calories: 180   Protein: 3 g   Carbohydrates: 19 g

Fat: 11 g   Sodium: 80 mg

13.3. Ricotta and Chocolate Chip Olive Oil Cookies

Prep Time: 15 minutes   Cooking Time: 25 minutes   Servings: 4

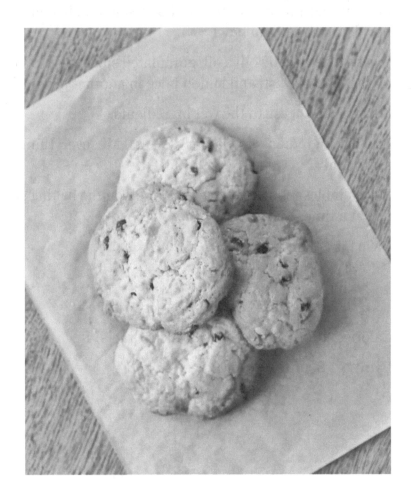

Ingredients

- 1 cup all-purpose flour
- ½ teaspoon baking powder
- ¾ cup granulated sugar

- ½ cup chocolate chips
- A pinch of salt
- ½ cup olive oil
- 1 large egg
- 1 teaspoon vanilla extract
- ½ cup ricotta cheese

Instructions

1. Heat oven to 350°F (180 °C). Line a baking sheet with parchment paper.
2. Combine all-purpose flour, nut flour, salt, and baking powder in a medium bowl.
3. Whisk together the olive oil, granulated sugar, egg, vanilla extract, and ricotta cheese in another bowl.
4. Add dry ingredients to wet ingredients. Mix everything thoroughly.
5. Add chocolate chips.
6. Take a tablespoon. Place the dough on the baking sheet one at a time.
7. Bake for 25 minutes.

Nutritional Information (per serving)

Calories: 220   Protein: 3 g   Carbohydrates: 26 g

Fat: 12 g   Sodium: 80 mg

13.4. Orange Ricotta Olive Oil Cookies

Prep Time: 15 minutes   Cooking Time: 25 minutes   Servings: 4

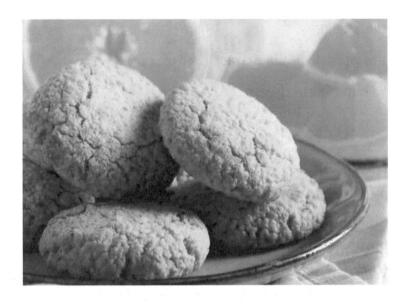

Ingredients

- 1 cup all-purpose flour
- ½ cup nut flour (or additional all-purpose flour)
- ½ teaspoon baking powder
- ½ cup olive oil
- ¾ cup granulated sugar
- 1 large egg
- 1 teaspoon vanilla extract
- 2 tablespoons fresh orange juice
- Zest of 1 orange
- ½ cup ricotta cheese
- A pinch of salt

1. Heat oven to 350°F (180 °C). Line a baking sheet with parchment paper.

2. Combine all-purpose flour, nut flour, salt, and baking powder in a medium bowl.

3. Whisk together the olive oil, granulated sugar, egg, vanilla extract, orange zest, and orange juice in a separate large bowl.

4. Add ricotta cheese to the wet ingredients.

5. Add dry ingredients to wet ingredients. Mix everything thoroughly.

6. Take a tablespoon and place the dough on the baking sheet one at a time.

7. Bake for 25 minutes.

Nutritional Information (per serving)

Calories: 180   Protein: 3 g   Carbohydrates: 19 g

Fat: 11 g   Sodium: 80 mg

13.5. Almond Olive Oil Cottage Cheese Cookies

Prep Time: 15 minutes   Cooking Time: 25 minutes   Servings: 4

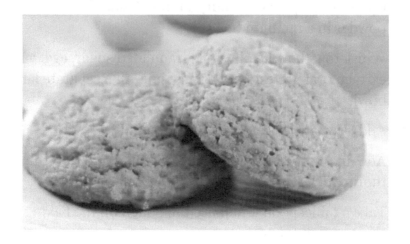

Ingredients

- ½ cup olive oil
- ½ cup granulated sugar
- ½ cup cottage cheese
- 1 large egg
- 1 teaspoon almond extract
- 2 cups all-purpose flour
- ½ teaspoon baking powder
- A pinch of salt
- Sliced almonds for topping

Instructions

1. Heat oven to 350°F (180 °C). Line a baking sheet with parchment paper.

2. Whisk together the olive oil, granulated sugar, cottage cheese, egg, and almond extract in a bowl.

3. Whisk the all-purpose flour, baking powder, and salt in another bowl.

4. Add dry ingredients to wet ingredients. Mix everything thoroughly.

5. Take a tablespoon and place the dough on the baking sheet one at a time.

6. Flatten each cookie and sprinkle sliced almonds on top.

7. Bake for 25 minutes.

Nutritional Information (per serving)

Calories: 190   Protein: 3 g   Carbohydrates: 24 g

Fat: 9 g   Sodium: 100 mg

13.6. Lemon Olive Oil Cake

Prep Time: 15 minutes   Cooking Time: 35 minutes   Servings: 4

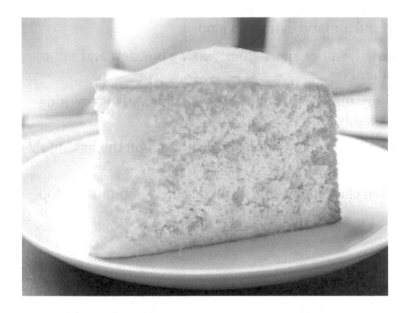

Ingredients

- 1 ½ cups all-purpose flour
- 1 cup granulated sugar
- 1 teaspoon baking powder
- ½ cup olive oil
- 2 large eggs
- 1 cup plain Greek yogurt
- Zest of 2 lemons
- 1 teaspoon vanilla extract
- A pinch of salt

Instructions

1. Heat oven to 350°F (180 °C). Take a 9-inch round cake pan. Brush it with olive oil. Sprinkle with flour.

2. Whisk the flour, sugar, baking powder, and salt in a bowl.

3. Whisk the olive oil, eggs, Greek yogurt, lemon zest, and vanilla extract in another bowl.

4. Add dry ingredients to wet ingredients. Mix everything thoroughly.

5. Pour the batter into the pie mold.

6. Bake in the oven for 35 minutes. Check for doneness with a toothpick.

Nutritional Information (per serving)

Calories: 350 Protein: 6 g Carbohydrates: 45 g

Fat: 16 g Sodium: 220 mg

13.7. Orange Almond Olive Oil Cake

Prep Time: 15 minutes   Cooking Time: 35 minutes   Servings: 4

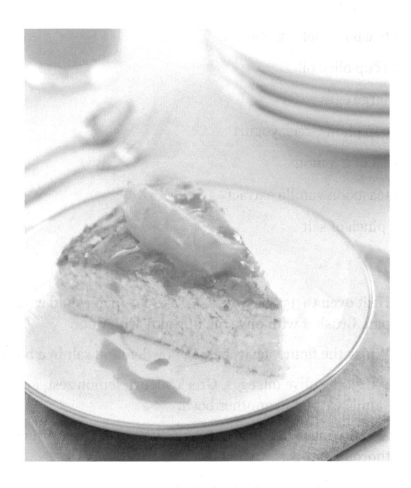

Ingredients

- 1 cup nut flour (or additional all-purpose flour)
- 1 cup all-purpose flour
- 1 cup granulated sugar
- 1 teaspoon baking powder
- ½ cup olive oil
- 2 large eggs
- ½ cup fresh orange juice
- Zest of 1 orange
- 1 teaspoon vanilla extracta
- A pinch of salt

Instructions

1. Heat oven to 350°F (180 °C). Take a 9-inch round cake pan and brush it with olive oil. Sprinkle with flour.

2. Combine the nut flour, all-purpose flour, sugar, baking powder, and salt in a bowl.

3. Whisk the olive oil, eggs, orange juice, orange zest, and vanilla extract in another bowl.

4. Add dry ingredients to wet ingredients. Mix everything thoroughly.

5. Pour the batter into the pie mold.

6. Bake in the oven for 35 minutes. Check for doneness with a toothpick.

Nutritional Information (per serving)

Calories: 380   Protein: 7 g   Carbohydrates: 45 g

Fat: 19 g   Sodium: 240 mg.

13.8. Vanilla Olive Oil Pound Cake

Prep Time: 15 minutes   Cooking Time: 45 minutes   Servings: 4

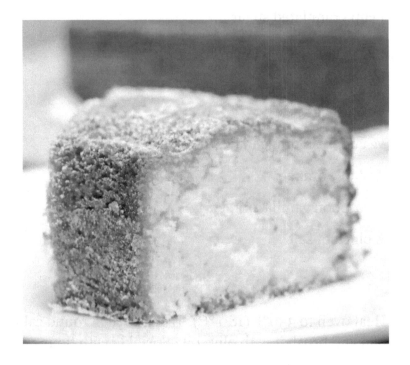

- 2 cups all-purpose flour
- 1 cup granulated sugar
- 1 teaspoon baking powder
- A pinch of salt
- 1 cup olive oil
- 3 large eggs
- 1 cup plain yogurt
- 1 tablespoon vanilla extract

Instructions

1. Heat oven to 350°F (180 °C). Take a 9-inch round cake pan, brush it with olive oil, and sprinkle with flour.
2. Mix flour, sugar, baking powder, and salt in a bowl.
3. Whisk together olive oil, eggs, yogurt, and vanilla extract separately.
4. Add dry ingredients to wet ingredients. Mix everything thoroughly.
5. Pour the batter into the loaf mold.
6. Bake in the oven for 45 minutes. Check for doneness with a toothpick.

Nutritional Information (per serving)

Calories: 420   Protein: 6 g   Carbohydrates: 45 g

Fat: 24 g   Sodium: 240 mg

Chapter 14:
Fish Dishes

14.1. Grilled Lemon-Herb Salmon

Prep Time: 15 minutes   Cooking Time: 10 minutes   Servings: 4

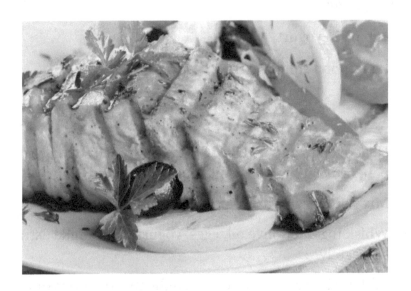

Ingredients

- 4 salmon fillets (about 1 lb)
- 2 tablespoons olive oil
- 1 tablespoon fresh lemon juice
- 1 teaspoon dried thyme
- Salt and pepper, to taste
- Cooked rice for serving
- Cooked grilled vegetables

Instructions

1. Preheat the grill to medium-high heat.
2. Whisk together olive oil, lemon juice, dried thyme, salt, and pepper in a bowl.
3. Brush the salmon fillets with this mixture.
4. Grill the fillets for 4–5 minutes per side.
5. Serve with cooked grilled vegetables and cooked rice.

Nutritional Information (per serving)

Calories: 300   Protein: 25 g   Carbohydrates: 2 g

Fat: 20 g   Cholesterol: 70 mg   Sodium: 150 mg

14.2. Salmon with Lemon-Dill Sauce

Prep Time: 10 minutes   Cooking Time: 10 minutes   Servings:4

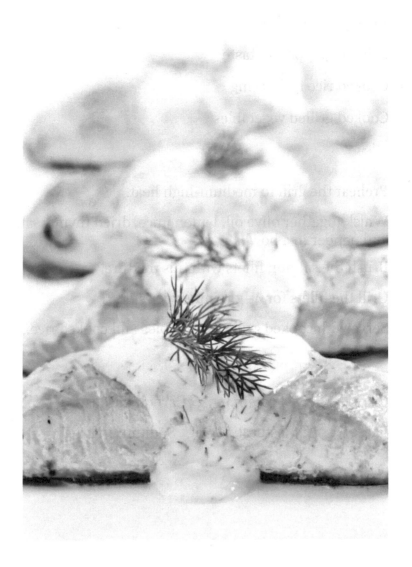

Ingredients

- 4 salmon fillets (about 1lb)
- 2 tablespoons olive oil
- 2 tablespoons fresh dill, chopped
- 1 teaspoon lemon juice
- Salt and pepper, to taste
- ½ cup Greek yogurt
- Cooked mashed potatoes for serving

Instructions

1. Season salmon fillets with salt and pepper.
2. Heat olive oil in a skillet over medium-high heat.
3. Place salmon fillets in the skillet, skin side down. Sear for 4–5 minutes. Sprinkle with salt and pepper. Turn the fillet over to the other side and cook for another 4–5 minutes.
4. Mix Greek yogurt, chopped dill, and lemon juice in a small bowl.
5. Serve with cooked mashed potatoes and lemon-dill sauce.

Nutritional Information (per serving)

Calories: 300 Protein: 30 g Carbohydrates: 3 g

Fat: 18 g Cholesterol: 80 mg Sodium: 90 mg

14.3. Avocado and Salmon Canapés

Prep Time: 15 minutes   Servings: 4

Ingredients

- 16 slices of cucumber
- 1 ripe avocado, sliced
- 4 ounces smoked salmon, thinly sliced
- Fresh chives, chopped, for garnish

Instructions

1. Slice the cucumber into 16 rounds.
2. Place an avocado slice on each cucumber slice.
3. Top with a slice of smoked salmon.
4. Garnish with chopped fresh chives.

Nutritional Information (per serving)

Calories: 120   Protein: 5 g   Carbohydrates: 6 g

Fat: 9 g   Cholesterol: 10 mg   Sodium: 150 mg

This page is for
YOUR NOTES

14.4. Baked Carp with Dijon Mustard

Prep Time: 15 minutes   Cooking Time: 30 minutes   Servings: 4

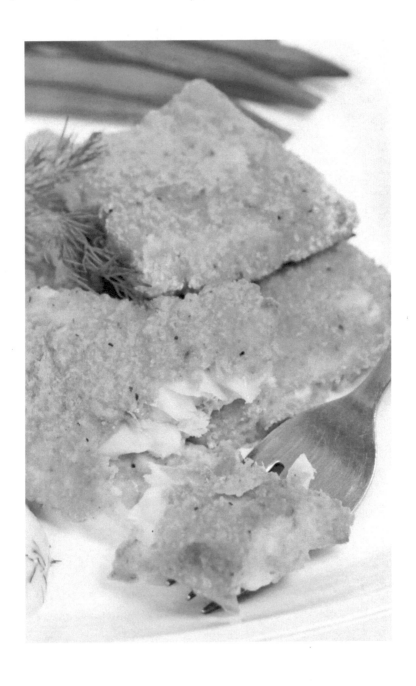

Ingredients

- 4 carp fillets about 1 lb
- 2 tablespoons Dijon mustard
- 1 tablespoon olive oil
- 1 cup breadcrumbs
- 2 cloves garlic, minced
- 1 teaspoon dried thyme
- Salt and pepper, to taste
- 1 cucumber sliced for garnish
- Cooked boiled potatoes for serving

Instructions

1. Preheat the oven to 400°F (200°C).
2. In a bowl, mix Dijon mustard and olive oil.
3. Combine breadcrumbs, minced garlic, dried thyme, salt, and pepper in another bowl.
4. Dip each carp fillet into the Dijon mixture, coating both sides.
5. Transfer the coated fillets to a baking sheet. Bake for 30 minutes.
6. Serve with cooked boiled potatoes and sliced cucumber.

Nutritional Information (per serving)

Calories: 250   Protein: 25 g   Carbohydrates: 15 g

Fat: 10 g   Cholesterol: 60 mg   Sodium: 350 mg

14.5. Carp with Vegetables in Tomato Sauce

Prep Time: 15 minutes   Cooking Time: 35 minutes   Servings: 4

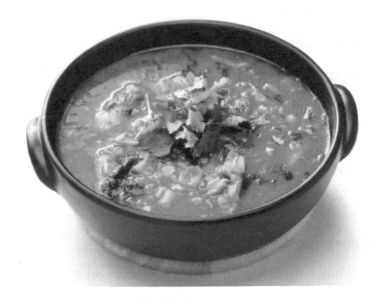

Ingredients

- 4 carp fillets about 1 lb

- 2 tablespoons olive oil

- 1 onion, finely chopped

- 3 cloves garlic, minced

- 2 bell peppers, thinly sliced

- 2 zucchinis, thinly sliced

- 1 can (28 oz) crushed tomatoes

- 1 teaspoon dried oregano

- 1 teaspoon dried basil

- Salt and pepper, to taste

Instructions

1. Sprinkle the carp fillet with salt and pepper, to taste.

2. In a large ovenproof skillet, heat the olive oil over medium-high heat. Cook the carp fillets for 2 minutes on each side. Remove from the pan to a plate.

3. Add chopped onion and minced garlic. Sauté in the same pan. Add the sliced bell peppers and zucchini. Cook for another 4 minutes.

4. Preheat the oven to 375°F (190°C).

5. Stir in the chopped tomatoes. Add the dried oregano, dried basil, salt, and pepper. Stir to combine. The sauce should simmer for 5 minutes.

6. Place the roasted carp fillets back into the skillet.

7. Transfer the pan to the preheated oven. Bake for 24 minutes.

Nutritional Information (per serving)

Calories: 340   Protein: 35 g   Carbohydrates: 25 g

Fat: 14 g   Cholesterol: 70 mg   Sodium: 800 mg

Chapter 15:
Meat Dishes

15.1. Beef Brisket Stew

*Prep Time: 15 minutes   Cooking Time: 1 ½ –2 hours
Servings: 4*

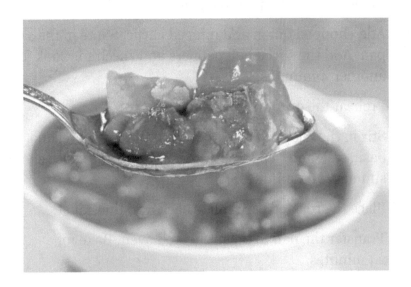

Ingredients

- 1 lb (450 g) beef brisket, cut into cubes
- 1 tablespoon vegetable oil
- 1 onion, diced
- 2 cloves garlic, minced
- 2 small carrots, peeled and sliced
- 2 potatoes, peeled and diced
- 2 cup water
- ¼ teaspoon black pepper coarse
- ¼ teaspoon cumin
- A pinch of cayenne pepper
- A pinch of nutmeg
- Salt, to taste

Instructions

1. Take a large pan. Heat vegetable oil in it over medium-high heat. Sear the beef brisket cubes until browned on all sides. Remove brisket from pan and place on a plate.

2. In the same pan, add onion and minced garlic. Sauté everything. Add carrots and potatoes. Cook for 3 minutes.

3. Return the seared brisket to the pot. Pour in water, add coarse black pepper, add salt and cumin, and stir.

4. Bring the stew to a boil. Then, reduce the heat to low. Cover and simmer for about 1 ½–2 hours or until the brisket is tender. When ready, add cayenne pepper and nutmeg.

Nutritional Information (per serving)

Calories: 200   Protein: 12.5 g   Carbohydrates: 15 g

Fat: 10 g   Cholesterol: 35 mg   Sodium: 400 mg

15.2. Beef Ribeye Stew

Prep Time: 15 minutes   Cooking Time: 1 ½–2 hours

Servings: 4

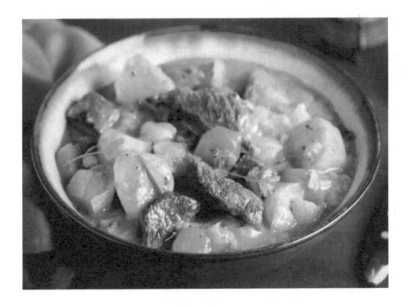

Ingredients

- 1 lb (450 g) beef ribeye, cut into cubes
- 1 tablespoon vegetable oil
- 1 onion, diced
- 2 cloves garlic, minced
- 2 small carrots, peeled and sliced
- 2 potatoes, peeled and diced
- 2 cup water
- ¼ teaspoon black pepper coarse

- A pinch of cayenne pepper

- 1 teaspoon dried thyme

- Salt, to taste

1. Take a large pan and heat vegetable oil in it over medium-high heat. Sear the beef ribeye cubes until browned on all sides. Remove the ribeye from the pot to a plate.

2. Add chopped onion and minced garlic to the same pan and sauté. Add carrots and potatoes. Cook for 3 minutes.

3. Return the seared ribeye to the pot. Pour in water, add coarse black pepper, add salt thyme, and stir.

4. Bring the stew to a boil. Then, reduce the heat to low. Cover and simmer for 1 ½–2 hours or until the ribeye is tender. When ready, add cayenne pepper.

Nutritional Information (per serving)

Calories: 200   Protein: 12.5 g   Carbohydrates: 15 g

Fat: 10 g   Cholesterol: 35 mg   Sodium: 400 mg

15.3. Chicken Curry Thai

Prep Time: 15 minutes   Cooking Time: 40 minutes   Servings: 4

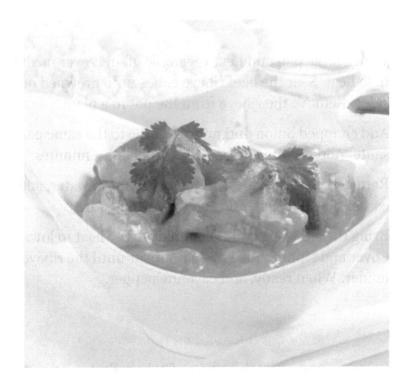

Ingredients

- 1 lb (450 g) chicken thighs without bones and skin. Cut them into pieces.
- 2 tablespoons vegetable oil
- 1 onion, finely chopped
- 3 cloves garlic, minced
- 1 tablespoon ginger, grated
- 2 tablespoons curry paste red or 1 tablespoon curry paste green
- 1 can (14 oz) coconut milk

- 1 cup water
- 1 bell pepper, sliced
- Salt and pepper, to taste
- Fresh cilantro for garnish
- Cooked rice for serving

Instructions

1. Take a large saucepan and heat vegetable oil in it over medium-high heat. Sauté the chicken pieces on all sides. Add chopped onion. Cook for 1 minute.

2. Prepare crushed garlic and grated ginger. Add to the pan. Add curry paste and stir. Pour in coconut milk and water. Stir well. Bring the curry to a boil. Then, reduce the heat to medium.

3. Add sliced bell pepper. Simmer over low heat for about 35 minutes. The chicken should become soft.

4. Season the curry dish with salt and pepper to taste. Garnish with cilantro. Serve the chicken curry over cooked rice.

Nutritional Information (per serving)

Calories: 250   Protein: 15 g   Carbohydrates: 10 g

Fat: 17.5 g   Cholesterol: 40 mg   Sodium: 450 mg

15.4. Chicken Curry Indian

Prep Time: 15 minutes   Cooking Time: 40 minutes   Servings: 4

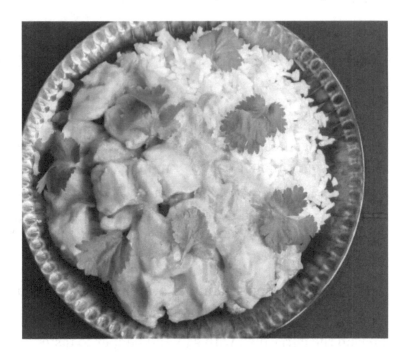

Ingredients

- 1 lb (450 g) chicken thighs without bones and skin. Cut them into pieces.
- 1 tablespoon vegetable oil
- 1 onion, finely chopped
- 2 cloves garlic, minced
- 1 teaspoon ginger, grated
- 1 tablespoon curry powder

- 1 cup coconut milk
- 1 cup water
- Salt and pepper, to taste
- Fresh cilantro for garnish
- Cooked rice for serving

Instructions

1. Take a large saucepan. Heat vegetable oil in it over medium-high heat. Sauté the chicken pieces on all sides. Add chopped onion. Sauté for 1 minute.

2. Prepare crushed garlic and grated ginger. Add to the pan. Add curry powder. Sauté 1 minute.

3. Pour in coconut milk and water. Stir well. Bring the curry to a boil. Reduce heat to medium.

4. Simmer over low heat for about 35 minutes. The chicken should become soft.

5. Season the curry dish with salt and pepper, to taste. Garnish with fresh cilantro. Serve the chicken curry over cooked rice.

Nutritional Information (per serving)

Calories: 225   Protein: 12.5 g   Carbohydrates: 15 g

Fat: 12.5 g   Cholesterol: 50 mg   Sodium: 400 mg

15.5. Pork Neck Meatballs

Prep Time: 15 minutes   Cooking Time: 15 minutes   Servings: 4

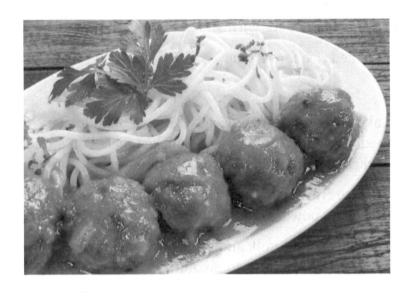

Ingredients

- ½ lb (225 g) ground pork neck
- 1 small caramelized onion
- ¼ cup breadcrumbs
- ¼ cup grated Parmesan cheese
- 1 egg
- 2 cloves garlic, minced
- Salt and pepper, to taste
- A pinch of cayenne pepper

- A pinch of nutmeg

- Olive oil for cooking

- Cooked pasta

- Cooked marinara sauce

Instructions

1. Combine ground pork neck, breadcrumbs, Parmesan cheese, egg, minced garlic, caramelized onion, cayenne pepper, nutmeg, salt and pepper in a bowl. Mix until well combined.

2. Using your hands, shape the mixture into small meatballs.

3. Heat the olive oil in a skillet over medium heat. Cook the meatballs for 10–15 minutes, turning occasionally, until browned and cooked.

4. Serve with cooked pasta and marinara sauce.

Nutritional Information (per serving)

Calories: 175 Protein: 10 g Carbohydrates: 5 g

Fat: 12.5 g Cholesterol: 55 mg Sodium: 250 mg

15.6. Marinara Sauce

Prep Time: 5 minutes   Cooking Time: 20 minutes   Servings: 2

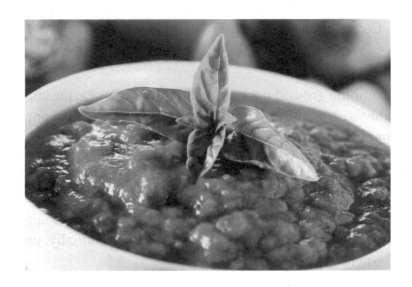

Ingredients

- 1 can (14 oz) crushed tomatoes
- 2 cloves garlic, minced
- 2 tablespoons olive oil
- 1 teaspoon dried oregano
- 1 teaspoon dried basil
- ½ teaspoon sugar (optional)
- Salt and pepper, to taste
- Crushed red hot pepper flakes (optional for heat)
- Fresh basil for garnish (optional)

Instructions

1. Heat the olive oil in a skillet over medium heat. Add minced garlic and sauté for about 1 minute. Be careful not to let it brown.

2. Pour in the crushed tomatoes. Stir well.

3. Add dried oregano, basil, sugar, salt, pepper, and crushed red hot pepper flakes.

4. Bring the sauce to a gentle simmer. Reduce the heat to low and let it simmer for 15–20 minutes.

5. Garnish with fresh basil if desired.

Nutritional Information (per serving)

Calories: 120   Protein: 3 g   Carbohydrates: 12 g

Fat: 7 g   Sodium: 300 mg

15.7. Meatballs with Ricotta

Prep Time: 15 minutes   Cooking Time: 15 minutes   Servings: 4

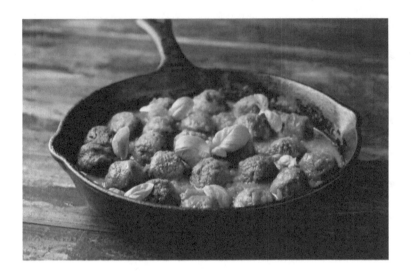

Ingredients

- ½ lb (225 g) ground pork neck
- ¼ cup ricotta cheese
- 2 tablespoons breadcrumbs
- ¼ cup grated Parmesan cheese
- 1 egg
- 2 tablespoons chopped fresh basil
- Salt and pepper, to taste
- Olive oil for cooking
- Cooked pasta
- Cooked marinara sauce

Instructions

1. Combine ground pork neck, ricotta cheese, breadcrumbs, Parmesan cheese, egg, chopped basil, salt, and pepper in a bowl. Mix until well combined.

2. Using your hands, shape the mixture into small meatballs.

3. Heat the olive oil in a skillet over medium heat. Cook the meatballs for 10–15 minutes, turning occasionally, until browned and cooked.

4. Serve with cooked pasta and marinara sauce.

Nutritional Information (per serving)

Calories: 180   Protein: 9 g   Carbohydrates: 5 g

Fat: 12.5 g   Cholesterol: 65 mg   Sodium: 300 mg

15.8. Grilled Lemon Herb Pork Ribs

Prep Time: 10 minutes   Cooking Time: 30–40 minutes

Servings: 4

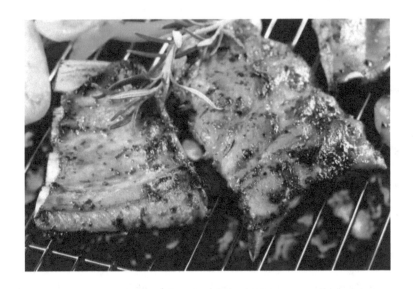

Ingredients

- 1 lb (450 g) pork ribs
- 1 tablespoon lemon juice
- 2 tablespoons olive oil
- 1 teaspoon dried thyme
- 1 teaspoon dried rosemary
- Salt and pepper, to taste
- Cooked grilled vegetables
- Cooked rice

Instructions

1. Cut the ribs into serving-size portions.
2. Mix lemon juice, olive oil, dried thyme, rosemary, salt, and pepper in a bowl. Coat the ribs with this mixture and let them marinate for at least 15 minutes.
3. Preheat the grill to medium-high heat. Grill the ribs for 15–20 minutes per side or until cooked through.
4. Serve with cooked grilled vegetables and cooked rice.

Nutritional Information (per serving)

Calories: 275 Protein: 10 g Carbohydrates: 5 g

Fat: 22.5 g Cholesterol: 45 mg Sodium: 75 mg

Conclusion

This is not just a cookbook; it's an invitation to the world of self-care and delicious discoveries.

I sincerely hope that every recipe and every piece of advice in this book becomes more than just.

Cooking— that it becomes a step toward better health and genuine pleasure from every meal.

Experiment, enjoy, create your culinary masterpieces, and take care of yourself.

There is much you can do to manage your condition and enhance the quality of your life, ultimately feeling more comfortable overall.

This page is for
YOUR NOTES

27568599R00080